Nothing

is Promised

By Marjorie E. Belson

To Ryan,
All the Best

Maj

Nothing is Promised

Interior Book Design and Layout by
www.integrativeink.com

ISBN: 978-0-9903888-0-7

Acknowledgments

Life often propels us to places unplanned and un-expected. My cancer was both unplanned and unexpected, but I was fortunate to have had access to excellent medical care and the support of both a wonderful family and kind, generous friends.

My army of doctors—Daniel Foitel, Mark Sultan, Alison Estabrook, Michael Grossbard, Joseph Finklestein, and their respective staff members—treated not only my body but in many ways also ministered to my soul. Being wrapped in their care allowed me to hope I would be well.

My most special thanks go to Matthew and Jodi. You continue to inspire me each day. To Maxie and Mutt, I can't quite forgive you both for having died. Larger than life, I expected you to live forever. To my grandchildren, Noah and Ariel, you are the future.

To my editor Karen Bartelt, for your faith in my abilities as a writer. To Thomas Curtis, my very capable graphic designer, for your tenacity and shared sense of humor. To Kevin Schwartz, my publicist, for tying up the loose ends.

To my wonderful husband Mel. Thank you for your unwavering love and dedication to me. I am truly whole.

Preface

I take comfort in the belief that our experiences can often set us free from our self-imposed constraints. My experiences led me to become the person I have always wanted to be—joyful in spirit and clear of purpose. It is a gift to be treasured prudently.

I am an ordinary person, special only to myself and to those who value me and would mourn my body's passage from this earth. I am one who has fought to overcome the limitations of her corporeal self and who can now acknowledge her strength.

Even though I have found my power, my mind is split in half. One side is joyful, full of endless hope and promise; the other shuns the light and overflows with fear and doubt. Always in conflict, it is a continuing struggle, as each side waits to claim me.

Initially, writing a memoir did not make me feel better because I so wished that its story was not mine to share. But having completed my work, I recognize that it has become a present to me, a way to embrace and validate my humanity, and an opportunity to encourage others to continue on their own journeys with strength and hope.

CONTENTS

December 2000 – June 2001
In An Instant 1

Pig On A Spit 6

Needle Localization: Crossing West 58th 10

Need To Know 14

Atlantic City 23

Diagnosis: Invasive Breast Cancer 29

Dr. S 36

Choices 38

The Assignment 43

Italy 48

August 1, 2001
Pre-Op 54

Night 59

August 2, 2001
Ambushed 60

Curtain Up 62

Recovery Room 65

Step Together 72

Caravan 76

Return 83

Reunion 1 89

Gone Missing 95

Drains 102

Oncologist 106

September 11, 2001
Back to Work 110

September 18, 2001 – June 2004
Lockdown 122

Cocktails 130

Trains 132

Something to Smile About 136

Implants 142

Restart 153

Dinner at Seven 160

Not Summer Camp 172

Return 2 182

CHAPTER ONE

December 2000 – June 2001
In An Instant

I walked into the darkened room to see a mass of black and white confusion clamped onto a backlit screen. Standing firm before these images, a radiologist. Pointing to finite changes in my left breast, he declared them to be neither age appropriate calcifications nor obvious cysts. Each needed to be examined by a breast surgeon immediately.

Sensing I was about to descend into hell, I could all but keep myself from collapsing. Crushed and alone, I felt frightened and trapped in the shadows of a limitless pit. Imagining cancer snaking around me forced me to focus on my end of days. At the prospect of having cancer, my breathing slowed, and my body felt like ice. Pulling my coat close gave me no relief from the chill. Numb, I walked back to the reception area to wait for copies of my errant mammograms to take to my surgeon for review.

Oblivious to much of the activity around me, I sat thinking about how quickly life changes. Just two weeks before, I'd danced at my son Matthew's wedding. Elegant in a floor length gown, I alone had walked him down the aisle, as his father had died years before. Tearful but strong, I rejoiced in his happiness as a witness to his vows and confident in his ability to build a life with his bride.

A wonderful party had followed, but by 2:00 a.m., I could laugh and dance no more. With shoes in hand, I'd returned to the stillness of my room, bowed my head, and sunk deep down into the folds of my gown to bless the newlyweds with peace, joy and good health. There was no warning that soon I'd be on my knees again, praying for my own good health.

For years, my mother-in law Maxie and I had scheduled our yearly mammograms together. As we waited for our test results, anxious to be cleared and on our way to lunch, we'd make silly, nervous conversation. Because of the excitement surrounding my son's wedding, we'd not scheduled our tests at the same time.

As the mother of Maxie's firstborn grandchild, she and I had remained more than close, even though her son and I had divorced many years before. Sharing up times and down, we'd become partners in gentle crimes. Much to the surprise and jealousy of some, our bond remained a testament to our love and respect for each other.

Today there would be no small talk, no sighs of relief, no Maxie shouting, "They damn near killed me. Let's get out of here. I want to eat and then go shopping." Instead, I'd awakened that morning with a premonition that without each other, one of us would not be well.

Seated in the crowded waiting area, I flipped nervously through a *People* magazine and thought I heard Maxie's distinctive voice. Seeing no one, I picked up the magazine again, believing it to be little more than my wish for her comfort.

Shortly thereafter I heard my name called again, but this time, it was too loud, too clear to be ignored. Visually tracking the sound, I watched Maxie stride across the busy waiting room until she stopped directly in front of me and planted her feet six inches from mine.

Our usual greeting was one of hugs and kisses, but today we remained stiff and distant. Without asking, she tossed aside the coat of some unknown person from the seat nearest to me and sat down in its place.

At 80 years of age, she remained a beautiful, colorful dynamo. Fierce in her loyalties, she was forever direct and clear. Though she believed "you can't fix stupid," she demanded to be heard and her positions considered.

She quickly explained that she'd come to get copies of her own mammograms, which were taken the day before and needed to be reviewed by our breast surgeon.

She said, "They saw a tiny spot on my right breast, and they're not sure what it is, or if it's anything at all. Damn it, we spend all this money for a mammography only to be told that they have no clue as to what they see when they see it." Almost as an afterthought she demanded, "Why the fuck are you here?"

Not knowing what kind of mood she was in, I took a deep breath and answered, "My mammography was not clear. I need to meet with the breast surgeon as soon as possible."

She closed her eyes, took my hand, squeezed it gently and said, "You're too little to have breast cancer."

At five feet two and a half inches, I was slim, well proportioned and enjoyed a modest 34-B bosom, but I knew that cancer could and would attack anyone without discrimination. Maxie's pronouncement was little more than her wish to keep me well. After waiting a few more long minutes, Maxie and I left the radiology center with copies of our x-rays and headed across town to learn our fate.

The surgeon's office was housed in a huge art deco building on the West Side of Manhattan. Once inside the doctor's high-tech suite, we handed the copies of our mammograms to the receptionist and followed her directions for preparing to be examined.

Too anxious to be separated, we squeezed ourselves into a changing booth for one and promptly fell on top of each other. After some awkward twists and turns, we emerged triumphant, each of us wearing paper-thin examination robes.

Our victory proved short lived.

Maxie was fine.

I was not.

To test the suspicious area in my left breast, I would undergo a stereotactic biopsy. Although the doctor tried to reassure me that all would be well, in that instant, I knew that I had breast cancer.

A profound sense of sadness pulled me deep into myself. It was an intuitive response that bored into my gut, tunneled inside my brain, and reached down to choke my heart.

This feeling was not based on negativity or despair, but rather on my recognition that one is often powerless to escape what one fears the most and that good health and longevity are not certainties. My mind fractured into snippets of words strung together, small exchanges spewed forth simultaneously, in rapid-fire between me and God, and me and me.

To Him, I expressed appreciation for my blessings: a healthy child, good family, great friends and a successful career. Although I very much wanted to live to see my yet-to-be-conceived grandchildren and revel in the delight of a private, personal, unconditional love, I accepted the timing of my illness, cognizant that so many had passed before me with lives abbreviated by pain and suffering.

At age 55, I could not truthfully say that my life would be cut short if I were to die from breast cancer, but very much wanting to live, my appeal to Him was to spare me from death and give me an alleviation from the terror I experienced, as I sought a rationale that would relieve me from having to accept responsibility for my cancer.

Questioning what, if anything, I was entitled to enjoy within my lifetime, I concluded that as both family and religion are accidents of birth, much else is just luck. No one is guaranteed anything. Simplified, cancer is not reflective of failure, but rather a terrible misfortune of life.

CHAPTER TWO

Pig On A Spit

During a stereotactic breast biopsy, small samples of tissue are removed from the breast using a vacuum-assisted needle guided to the correct location via x-rays and computer coordinates. This information did nothing to prepare me for mine, which took place one week after having seen my breast surgeon.

Directed to a remote section of the hospital, I changed from my street clothes into a hospital gown, and then walked into the adjoining room where I would undergo my procedure. Inside, a strange looking table was anchored next to an impressive machine with a large, open screen.

A technical assistant stood in front of this equipment. Seated to her left at a worn, ordinary desk was the doctor. A small, gnome-like woman, she was hunched over some forms and waved me to the table without looking up. Speaking more to herself than to me, she mumbled, "Your procedure will be over shortly. It should not cause you much discomfort. My assistant will tell you when I am ready."

Less than perfunctory, this doctor was rude. My instincts warned me to leave before she cut into my breast, but as I moved to the door, she lifted her head and said, "Where are you going? I'm ready for you now."

I very much wanted to leave, but my need to confirm that I did have cancer took precedence. When instructed to climb onto an unforgiving table and lay face down on its cold surface, I did.

As I strained to place my left breast through the opening beneath me, the hard platform bruised my skin, which made it difficult for me to angle it into the gaping hole. Lying painfully on my collarbone, the technician's hands pulled and prodded my small breast until it was in place. With minimal counsel, the opening shut with a loud snap and locked my breast in position. Exposed and trapped in a vise, I wanted the doctor to be quick and accurate. She proved to be neither.

Without further delay, a long, thin wire with a pincer-shaped knife at its tip cut deep into my breast. Pain radiated throughout my body, each thrust of the knife more agonizing than its precursor. With a ferocity equal to that of a coal miner desperately seeking to make his day's quota, the doctor hacked at my breast. Wanting to rip my body free, I tried to pull up from the table, but fastened in place, I was powerless. Utterly defenseless, I felt much like a pig impaled on a spit.

I screamed at the doctor, begging her to stop, or at the very least numb the area, but relentless in her task, she burrowed still further into my body and muttered, "Tissue samples need to be cut as quickly as possible. I have no time to waste with administering anesthesia."

I cried out, "I'm your damn patient, and I'm in too much unnecessary pain. Give me something now. You're killing me." She said nothing.

After one last angry plunge of her knife, the doctor withdrew her weapon from my breast. Freed from the table's grip, I crawled off dripping blood onto the floor. Given bandages by the assistant, I covered my wounds, dressed quickly, and left the office without a word.

Outside, I steadied myself against the hospital's cold brick wall and breathed in the chilly December air. Disconnected, weak and vulnerable, I watched the crush of New Yorkers pass by me. Inwardly, I raged against the brutality of the day's procedure and wished I'd let Maxie come with me, for at the very least, she'd have pulled me off that table and all but beat on the doctor before security was called.

Today's experience had been awful, the doctor beyond cruel. The lack of communication between us enraged me. Was it necessary to endure a pain so intense? Never again would I allow myself to be subjected to either physical or psychological brutality.

Perhaps I was one of too many patients and that validated the decision to not waste time with an analgesic. Perhaps the doctor had overbooked her schedule. Perhaps the doctor reveled in having total control over my body and relished inflicting pain.

A cyst was found behind the nipple of my left breast, and it would need to be removed. However, steadfast in my belief that I did have cancer, this news did not allow me to rest easy.

CHAPTER THREE

Needle Localization: Crossing West 58ᵗʰ

My cyst had to be removed surgically, and Maxie and I were not at all pleased. Specifically, a wire would be inserted via a hollow needle into my breast to localize the metal clip placed there during my stereotactic biopsy.

I could only think that barbarians would next be at my chest, poised to skewer me with sharp instruments, salivating repulsively as they anticipated my pain. Then, off I would go to the operating room to have the tissue removed and evaluated. At least I would be given drugs for pain and induced into a much needed, sedated sleep.

Maxie debated with me as to how much time I would take off from my job as a pre-school teacher and whether I would recuperate at her home. I thought two days of rest in my own home would be sufficient.

Unsurprisingly, Maxie disagreed with my plan. "You're so damn independent. You should stay at my house with me for a week. You must like to drive me nuts with worry."

"Maxie, I love you for caring and even more for being annoyed—okay, angry—with me." I shrugged my shoulders and continued, "I just need to be able to tune out."

Maxie softened and unexpectedly, answered, "Marjorie, I do understand how you feel, and I do respect your wishes, but I hate to see you alone at home."

"I'm really okay, and you and Matthew are nearby. Thank you."

Ah, but if only my needle biopsy had gone as smoothly as I defined it. But definitions are just textbook explanations, impersonal conclusions not always applicable in the real world. Humans control machines, and both machines and humans have low ends to their bell curves of performance. My procedure proved to be a challenge.

While Maxie stewed in the waiting room, anxious for my latest commotion to be over, I changed into a robe, opened it at the waist, spread my legs and straddled the mammography machine, which allowed my left breast to be secured in place.

Working from the monitoring screen, the doctor gave the technician the coordinates to mark the subject tissue with the hollow needle and insert a wire to pinpoint the area to be removed. Each thrust was recorded on the monitor, each stab was felt and repeated until the needle had found its mark: the metal clip inserted at the time of my stereotactic biopsy.

Feeling wet, I looked down. Blood gushed from my breast, and I wanted to puke, but instead, I asked for ice chips to suck on while the red surge was staved with a compression bandage. Soon after, the radiologist remarked that she'd found another spot, which she thought should be screened.

Lovely, more prods and pokes.

My left breast rebelled and tried to duck another jab, but it was down for the count. I was a standing target, seated. The needle hit the mark somewhere midway between the left nipple and left armpit, and victory was declared.

With wires taped against my breast, I was wrapped with a second examination robe, placed in a wheelchair and sent to roll and rock across West 58th Street with two attendants (one to push me and one to carry my file). Maxie led the charge to the surgical suite across the street.

To cross West 58th on a good day was tricky, but this was totally insane, as I became part of a motley troop of prime targets lined up on the curb, waiting to get to the other side of the street without being killed during midday New York City traffic.

To my left, a man sat in a wheelchair. To my immediate right was a very pregnant woman with three children at hand. Next to her were two adults, one with a cane and another with a walker. Without divine intervention, none of us had a chance to navigate safely to the other side.

Directly across the thoroughfare, I could see the entrance to the hospital's emergency room. It was easy to imagine the many pedestrians, all of them victims of failed attempts to cross this street, carted there for resuscitation and re-stitching.

Our divine intervention came quickly and in the form of Maxie. As she murmured, "I know you can't fix stupid, but this is beyond stupid," she stepped off the curb into the street. Smartly dressed as ever, with her Hermes handbag held high, she waved it dramatically over her head, then stopped in the middle of the block and challenged each driver to pass her.

Horns blew, brakes screeched, bicyclists shouted obscenities, but no matter, she was not to be intimidated. In a moment, all traffic on West 58th Street stopped; it was a New York miracle.

Those of us who'd been desperate to cross the street shouted, clapped, banged walkers, raised canes, and cheered their approval at her courage. With a royal flick of her wrist, Maxie turned to wave us across West 58th Street. I laughed so hard that the needles shook in my breast.

Once again, victory was short-lived. Although the cyst was clean and the other tissue sample resulted in a diagnosis of non-invasive breast cancer, I remained convinced that invasive breast cancer had tiptoed into my body.

CHAPTER FOUR

Need To Know

Ripping through New York City's rush hour traffic with a diagnosis of non-invasive breast cancer psychologically strapped to my chest, I was impatient to garage my car, sprint inside my apartment and sift through my jumbled emotions without distraction.

Eager to make both professional and personal changes in my life, I'd thought that the calm after my son's wedding would be a perfect time for me to explore my options, but after meeting with my doctor that afternoon, I wondered if I had any future at all.

In record time, I dashed into my apartment too wired, too anxious to take pleasure in its predictable console. Decorated in an eclectic mix of fabric and furniture, my home was warm and colorful. Until that moment, it had been my still, safe place.

Within minutes, my phone rang.

My first reaction was to wonder if the angel of death was calling me, even though I had an unlisted telephone number, but then again bad news does find you no matter what safeguards are created.

The phone rang again, and again.

I answered.

An unfamiliar voice identified herself as a breast cancer survivor and a volunteer from the Breast Cancer Center. With ill-repressed delight, she informed me that she'd be available to answer any questions about my cancer and that I'd "become a sister within a very special group of cancer patients for whom there were myriad classes dedicated to my health and well being."

She ended her litany of goods and services with "You should be thankful for the good news as to the type of cancer you have."

Speechless, I just glared at the phone.

My privacy had just been hijacked, outsourced to a bizarre, invisible space where support was scripted. Though I appreciated any information regarding my health, I was appalled by this stranger's insensitivity to me. She was a negative intrusion into my life and one whom I sensed took pleasure in me joining her "sisterhood."

How could she, or anyone else, make a pronouncement as to how I should react to my diagnosis of cancer? Not having any cancer at all would be good news. I certainly didn't feel special and was far too reserved for instant intimacies. "We both have cancer, let's do lunch," did not work for me.

My answer, "Thank you, goodbye."

To protect myself from the insensitivity of others, I would need to be circumspect in my choice of confidants, for though people are often moved by others' difficulties, it is rare that they will experience a permanent shift in their attitudes beyond the moment. Support for me would best come from those I trusted, not from strangers.

Among my family and friends, who could give me the solace I would surely need? Perhaps a game—"Do I Trust You With My Feelings?"—would be the way to go. The only prize would be a ticket to my life, which at the moment was not a terrifically happy one.

After some consideration, I decided who qualified to be contestants.

1. Maxie: Tough call.

To share my thoughts and concerns with a woman who'd endured the loss of one child and the disabilities of another was difficult. In all but denial of my diagnosis, she tried her best to will my cancer away. Nonetheless, she remained a source of consolation and humor.

Maxie answered my phone call in singular form. "Where the hell have you been? What did the doctor say? You don't have breast cancer. I just don't understand all the commotion."

"Maxie, I have non-invasive breast cancer and need to be monitored to see if I develop invasive breast cancer."

"Oh crap," was her reply before she slammed her phone down and ended our conversation.

Within minutes, Maxie was back on the line, subdued. She said softly, "I'm sorry, I didn't expect your news. I still don't believe it. Tests are often wrong." Then she added, "Please tell me what I can do for you."

"Just stay calm. I'm in good hands," I replied.

2. Matthew and Jodi: Keep it clear and positive.

Collectively and individually, my son and daughter-in-law are the brightest and kindest of people; they complemented each other beautifully. With her compassion and consideration, Jodi had expanded the circle of our family.

He a journalist, she a midwife, they were a stunning couple. Each radiated a fierce energy, and together they projected formidable power. Young and strong, they were ready and eager to face life as partners.

I dreaded telling them that I was not well, for as parents, we hope to spare our children all that is difficult or hurtful in life, yet sadly there are times when we ourselves become that from which we so desperately want to protect them. Nonetheless, as my relationship with them was predicated on honesty, I could not consider anything else.

Seated in their living room, I shared with Matthew and Jodi the results of my biopsies. Their concern for my health was palpable, as anxious, sad expressions quickly replaced their smiles. Jodi moved from her chair to sit next to me on the couch and hugged me tight, while Matthew stood up, sighed heartbreakingly deep and said, "Oh no." Then he walked behind me, put his hands on my shoulders, and kissed the top of my head.

When Jodi asked the first question, "Will your cancer become invasive?" Matthew returned to his chair and faced me.

Looking from one to the other, I said quietly, "I need to be watchful. I have no guarantees that it will or will not."

"Mom, what can you do to prevent it?" said Matthew.

"Who really knows? Maybe diet, or maybe exercise. Frankly, the best thing for me to do is to try to calm my nerves and make cancer disappear into the back of my mind so that I can get through each day without being scared to death."

"What can we do?" Matthew asked.

"Nothing. Well yes, there is something to do. Let's belly up to a bar and get ourselves some stiff drinks on me."

"Great idea. Second round on me," Jodi said, as we walked out their front door.

3. Best girlfriends Ava and Marlo: Remain vibrant and optimistic.

Breast cancer strikes too close to women for them to digest news of a friend's diagnosis comfortably. It is a psychological jolt that calls into question one's own mortality. It's a frightening disease whose proximity can engender unspoken, unconscious recoil from imagined malignant cells.

With this in mind, I was more than a bit hesitant to drag them into my mess, but my two best friends would be furious with me if I didn't give them the chance to support me. Marlo and I agreed that we would meet for a snack. I spoke with Ava that same night. Although she'd just put her infant son to bed, Ava was eager to talk to me.

"Marjorie, how did you make out with your test the other day? The baby was sick and I didn't have a chance to call. He's been up for what seems like forever, but finally his fever broke, and he just went to sleep. I know that you're fine, but please say the words."

My response was too slow for her not to intimate that all was not well, so she shot back, "Okay, what's wrong?"

"I have non-invasive breast cancer, and I need to be watched closely."

"Oh no!" she shouted. "This makes no sense. You don't deserve it, and no one does. I can't believe that the possibility of developing invasive breast cancer will hang over you. I'm just so mad. What can I do?"

"Pray for me; get some rest."

"No," she shouted, "there has to be more."

"Ava. Right now, we just have to wait."

My conversation with Ava drained me emotionally. Some things are best left unsaid, but illness is often not a personal event when family and friends need to be considered. I didn't want to upset Marlo, but for me not to share with her my information would make me less of a friend.

She and I had a favorite restaurant in Dumbo, well within the shadows of the Brooklyn Bridge. Although it was midweek and ten o'clock at night, we were regulars, and the owner welcomed us: "I know just what you two ladies would like."

Our small table faced the bistro's small, well-lit patio. There, weeks before, Marlo and I had decided to vacation in Italy the following summer. Now I wondered if I would be able to go.

As soon as we'd sat down, Marlo whispered, "I know something is not right. You waited two days to call me since you took your tests. If the news had been good, you would've rung me up and shouted, 'I'm okay,' before you got back home, but you didn't. It wasn't fair to make me wait."

"Marlo, I'm sorry. I just didn't know what to say. I have non-invasive breast cancer, which sounds good, but deep down, I know that my body will fail me, and I'll be faced with invasive breast cancer."

Marlo let go of my hand, covered her face for a minute, then looked up at me and said, "I will pray for you and be ready to support you any way that you let me."

Made speechless by her kindness, I jumped up from the table, opened the door to the garden, and rushed outside. Marlo quickly followed me and put her arm around my waist to shield me from the cold wind. We stood side by side until the owner called us to dinner.

4. Mother: Tell nothing.

At the time, my mother was 90. Alert and reaching for 100, she was not emotionally equipped to deal with illness at any level. As a young girl, she'd cared for her cancer-stricken mother, who had died at age 43. Ever living in fear of disease, my mother would have been unable to comfort me. To continuously assuage her terror would have been more than I could possibly do. In truth, some things are best left unsaid.

5. Mutt: Tell everything, and omit nothing.

How we met was unimportant. That the friendship endured is what made it special. Two independents, our love and respect for each other had held fast over the years. As he'd survived a quintuple bypass, I knew that he, above all, would best understand how I felt about the tenuousness of my life and my disappointment in having reached a point of inner strength only to be cut down with breast cancer.

Mutt had all but insisted that he come with me to the doctor, but I wanted no distraction from my thoughts. Less than satisfied with my choice, he waited for my phone call.

"Baby Girl, just tell me that you're okay."

"I'm not quite perfect."

"Nonsense, you're more than perfect."

"Mutt, I have breast cancer. At this time it's non-invasive, but I just don't feel very good about this."

"What did you say? Your doctor is nuts. Let's find another doctor. I will find someone."

"Mutt, my doctor is fine. The tests are accurate. I just have to be monitored. It's going to drive me crazy. I'm scared..."

He interrupted me mid-sentence. "I will not have you get cancer on my watch." I heard him cough violently as he struggled to catch his breath.

"Mutt, please, calm down, otherwise I won't tell you anything. You have a heart condition. You will not drop dead on me."

After a few minutes of silence, he managed, "Okay, why don't we both check into a sanatorium by the sea? Wrapped in blankets, we could sit in the sun, be fed some grapes and cheese, finish off a bottle of wine and then make love."

"Mutt," I laughed, "you are ridiculous."

"I love you."

"Goodbye."

21

Mutt's fury at the fact that I could face a serious illness had been a welcome release for me. I'd dared not voice my own anger for fear of committing hubris and being struck down.

CHAPTER FIVE

Atlantic City

Though my health-care professionals were convinced that my prognosis was excellent, throughout the next six months I was neither happy nor reassured. How could I be?

There were no definitive answers, only statistical probabilities. Facing my surgically compromised left breast each day only underscored the unpredictability of my health.

Cancer had crept inside my body, but how? If I could find this out, perhaps I could better protect myself from yet another attack.

Better still, a sign would signal a cell's transition from benign to malignant. Perhaps the sign would be bells and whistles? Perhaps invasive breast cancer would whisper in my ear, "Hey Marjorie, gotcha."

To accept that the answers I needed were independent from my need to know and that they would reveal themselves in their own time both frustrated and sickened me, but I was impotent to do more.

Seeking a temporary release from my miserable thoughts, I dragged myself to a yoga class given weekly at the hospital for those battling cancer. I went to the session, apprehensive as to what my reaction would be when surrounded by other cancer patients.

Dimly lit and painted a depressing shade of gray, the studio was far from welcoming. The class participants remained stiff and silent. Each of them seemed intent on avoiding contact with the others, as if to do so might confirm their illnesses over and over again.

Still sore from my lumpectomies, I eased myself slowly down onto the narrow mat. Stretching my body into each position was difficult, so I compensated by limiting my movements. The unnatural quiet coupled with the physical coldness of the room made me feel as if we all were bloodless shadows, moving without grace, struggling to find an elusive peace.

I wondered, who among us would be the next to die?

I fled the class and never returned.

Long after the short ride home from yoga, I became more depressed and plunged from a state of passive acceptance into one of frenetic anxiety. My survival was now dependent on Ambien and frequent, joyless trips to Atlantic City.

Calmed by the open road, I sipped my coffee, listened to music and relished the privacy of my thoughts. For those few hours, I was free to feel whatever I wished, or better still, feel nothing at all.

Trips to Atlantic City had not always been devoid of joy. Years ago, Maxie had introduced me to the mixed charms of gambling. She played slot machines with abandon, anywhere and anytime she could. Atlantic City was close enough to our homes to make a day trip easily possible.

My passion to play began innocently enough. In need of a travel companion, Maxie asked me to take the ride with her to Atlantic City. Having nothing planned for that day, I said yes without any thought other than to bring with me a very small amount of money in order to play one machine.

That inaugural ride to Atlantic City was fun. As we made the trip there, Maxie provided me with a detailed tutorial on how to play slot machines and described the pros and cons of each machine in detail.

"Try to find the ones with triple payouts. The Lucky Sevens always hit. Do not play the 10 X Winnings, they rarely pay anything, and forget the Progressives; you're screwed."

"Remember," she said, "hot machines hit winners like crazy and crank out a pot of money. Cold machines have the potential of turning into winners, but whether to stay or leave, that's a crapshoot." It was free will at its worst.

Maxine's dissertation ended when we saw Atlantic City's skyline jut onto the horizon almost three hours later. As if a switch had been turned on, she began to think out loud as to which machine she would first play.

"Should it be the Gold Triple Bar? I cleaned up there last time. Or the Triple 7s to try to win back all the money I'd lost?" Maxie mulled over her choices until we left the car. Then she said, "I am going back to those Triple 7s and win back my money."

Although I felt much like an Olympic athlete whom Maxie had coached to bring home the gold, I was totally unprepared for the shock of the casino's gaming floor. The sounds of bells, whistles, shouts, and screams merged together with the nonstop hum of spinning roulette wheels and the rolling of dice.

The lights were dim, so it took time for my eyes to adjust and see hundreds of people arched over acres of slot machines and betting tables. Weaving between them were scantily dressed, leggy beverage ladies along with casino attendants, croupiers, and security. It was fabulous.

In short order, Maxie showed me where to put my quarters, pull the handle, or push the button on a quarter machine. Then she cautioned, "Drink lots of coffee. It's free, and you need to be alert. Be aware of the people around you, and keep your pocketbook closed." Then she kissed me good luck, spun on her heel, and took off to the other side of the casino without looking back.

My first pull graced me with three cherries in a row and multiplied my quarter by three. I was a winner and was hooked. It was that simple, that uncomplicated, and that much mindless fun.

After accumulating a stockpile of fifty dollars, rather than take my winnings and leave, I promptly put them back into what I had thought was my lucky machine. I lost it all.

Maxie found me reading in the lounge. Flush from play, she whispered, "I've won a great deal of money." Without hesitation, she reached into her bag and pulled out a huge stack of money. She quickly peeled off a large bill and handed it to me.

In a flash, I was back on the floor, feeling bold and now playing fifty-cent machines. After a slow start, things began to roll, and I quickly made back what Maxie had given me. This time, I took my spoils and left.

I started to return the money she'd staked me with, but she raised her hand and shook her head no. Then she laughed and said, "What is given is given."

Maxie had a personal driver at her disposal, and he would often drive us to Atlantic City. This was lovely, as she and I could relax and enjoy the ride. The dynamic between us changed little, though when we wished for our conversation not to be overheard by the chauffeur, we lowered our voices to a whisper, as if we were young girls telling each other secrets.

Food was an important component of our casino adventures. We usually stopped along the Garden State Parkway for a light brunch on our way to the Jersey Shore. As we preferred our own fare to fast food, we packed some snacks and stopped to eat them at the rest areas along the way.

We were quite the spectacle. Her uniformed driver walked directly behind Maxie and me carrying two shopping bags, one filled with food and the other paper goods. After finding an empty table, we sanitized it with handi-wipes, and then sat down to enjoy our rations.

I missed those carefree moments with Maxie, but now the thought of anyone's company was more than I could stand. Frightened at the thought of my cancer becoming invasive, conversation at any level would have been more than I could tolerate.

I started taking trips to the casino alone. The anonymity of the casino became the backdrop for my personal drama. Soothingly addictive, the spin of the slot machines' wheels seduced me into oblivion. Playing one machine at a time was never enough; two were a given, three was best. Whether I won or lost didn't matter. I felt no joy and craved no exchange, no counsel. My only goal: escape into the moment.

CHAPTER SIX

Diagnosis: Invasive Breast Cancer

Six months later, I underwent another mammography. To the surprise of everyone but me, I did not pass with flying colors and underwent another painful stereotactic biopsy.

A phone call informed me that indeed invasive breast cancer had been found in my left breast. In my right breast, there was so much suspect tissue that undergoing so many localizations would be pointless; any subsequent lumpectomies would all but eradicate its tissue.

Cancer had proven to be imperious; its entrance required no proclamations. Last time, breast cancer had taken me prisoner without a trial, now it was ready to execute me.

This news was not unexpected. I'd enjoyed less than perfect health for years. There had been too many surgeries, too many doctors and far too much pain. Just twelve months earlier I'd had a hysterectomy, and before that, joint replacements and a gangrened appendix, all in a relatively short span of time.

I was tired, but realizing that wondering which test would be "the one" would no longer torment me, I experienced a strange sensation of relief. For months, not knowing if I would develop invasive breast cancer had gnawed at my gut. Without a definitive "You will never fall prey to the disease" to reassure me, I'd become wary of my future.

The phone rang in the bedroom. I stared at it, hesitating to answer, anxious that this might signal more bad news, but having had more than my share that day, odds were this was a friendly call. I lifted the receiver to my ear.

It was my friend Mutt, who'd called to find out the results of my latest tests. When he heard my answer, "I've been diagnosed with invasive breast cancer," his response was an audible gasp.

His reaction pushed me to my emotional edge and forced my mind to wrap itself around the horrifying implications of invasive breast cancer. I hung up the phone.

Straightaway, the phone began to ring, again and again. Ignoring its screams, I turned it off. I'd had enough tests, diagnoses, surgeries, and long recuperations. I went to bed and wept.

Thirty minutes later, I heard a loud knock on my door. I reached for a robe and asked, "Who's there?"

"Me."

Speechless, I opened the door and collapsed into Mutt's arms. Guiding me into the living room, he sat me down next to him on the sofa. As I tried to describe my feelings, he placed his fingers on my lips. Between us, no explanation was needed. He knew that I'd not meant to push him away, but flooded with so much bad news, I'd needed to propel myself back from the water's edge to escape drowning. Secure with him near, I fell asleep in minutes.

With his body stretched against mine, he held me close throughout the remainder of that night. Feeling the warmth of my breath against his chest, I'd wished to linger there forever, cradled in his arms, savoring his scent, secure in his presence.

I'd cared for him forever, but to me, he'd always remained larger than life. Intimidated by his strength of purpose, I'd never shared my feelings with him, but lying next to him felt right. Huddled against him, I felt protected, out of harm's way—until the idea of my cancer punched my brain awake.

My health issues demanded that I focus all my attention on the conference with my surgeon, which would take place later that day.

Trying not to wake him, I unraveled my body from Mutt's arms and went into the den.

I turned on the computer to read material relevant to invasive breast cancer, but it quickly became an overload of medical data and too difficult for me to process. I powered down the computer and walked back to the living room, where I gently slid my body alongside Mutt's back. Relaxed, I fell asleep until he woke me with a kiss on my cheek.

He sat down next to me and said, "Baby Girl, I need to get back home to do some work, and you need to get ready for your appointment with your doctor. Are you sure you don't want me to go with you?"

"Thank you, no, but I'll imagine you in my back pocket."

"Just don't make me wait to hear from you."

"Promise."

It was time for him to leave and for me to shower and dress for my doctor's appointment, so I got up from bed and walked him to my front door, where he held me tight and whispered, "You have some big steps to take, but you can do it. Remember, I'm here for you." He kissed me again, opened the door and left.

Before I had time to be sad to see him go, the phone rang. It was Maxie.

Annoyed, she said, "You didn't call me yesterday; what is wrong?"

Her question was legitimate. We usually spoke to each other daily. Sometimes we talked at length, sometimes not. Often we tried to complete the *New York Times*' crossword puzzle together, but most of the time it was just the recap of our days and a shared laugh at something silly.

I updated her with my latest breast cancer development.

"Goddamn it" was her response. She asked when I would see the doctor.

I replied, "After I wash and dress, I will be on my way."

She said, "Okay," and abruptly hung up the phone.

The warm water ran over my body as I stood in the shower. I wished it were able to wash my cancer away, but it was useless, so I turned the water off and dried my body

with a soft, sweet smelling towel. I took extra care with my bosom and gently patted it dry.

Surgery and reconstruction would wreak havoc on my breasts. The violence I imagined caused me to shudder. I threw down the towel, dressed and walked to the garage to start my car and be off.

As the garage door opened, a familiar car blocked the driveway. There was Maxie, seated in the back of her car, her driver at the ready. I was astonished to see her sitting there. Not normally an early riser, for her to be dressed and out of her house before ten o'clock was impressive.

As I walked to her, she rolled down her window and commanded, "Park your car, and get in mine. You're not going to the doctor without me. Jodi will meet us there."

Speechless, I obeyed, relieved that she and Jodi would be with me that morning to meet with the doctor. I also hoped Maxie had already eaten something, or it would be a rather long ride to West 58th Street with a woman who was cranky because of a missed meal.

Seated in the surgeon's office, we represented three generations of our family, three perspectives on life, three pairs of ears to hear, three pairs of eyes to see, and three brains to absorb the information set before us.

I heard little and saw even less when showed the diagrams of what my surgery would entail. Cancer stayed close to my body and dared me to make it go away. For me to submit to another lumpectomy followed by a series of radiation treatments would not be acceptable. I wanted the cancer ripped from my body immediately, and I was determined to undergo a bilateral mastectomy and begin to reconstruct my breasts at the same time. I scheduled my bilateral mastectomy for August 2, 2001, less than six weeks away.

Ultimately, my surgery would consist of two parts. During the first half, my breast surgeon would remove all breast tissue, both nipples and any affected lymph nodes. During the second part, the reconstructive surgeon would cut my chest muscles vertically in half so tissue expanders, which looked like deflated balloons with an access port, could be placed inside the muscle.

I imagined my bilateral mastectomy would be similar to a tag team-wrestling match. In one corner of the operating theater would be my breasts, in the other would be the two surgeons dressed in matching blue scrubs with abstractly painted bandanas about their heads.

My breasts would be down for the count after the first doctor scooped out all their tissue. Finished, she would turn to the second surgeon and tag his hand. This would signal him to jump into my chest, cut its muscles, and pop tissue expanders inside.

Within four weeks after this surgery, saline would be injected into these expanders weekly in order to stretch my chest muscles to fit each breast cavity, thereby creating a natural contour and fluidity of motion. Upon reaching the desired size, implants would be inserted into the newly enlarged chest muscles. In time, I hoped both my breasts and I would heal, and together we would spring back to life and be on top of our game.

With nothing more to do, Maxie, Jodi, and I then thanked the patient doctor for her time and made our way to the street. As we waited together on the corner of Ninth Avenue and West 58th for the driver to pick us up, Maxie, Jodi, and I gathered each other up for a poignant group hug that ended when Maxie declared, "I don't know about you, but I'm hungry. Let's go eat lunch."

CHAPTER SEVEN

Dr. S

The next day, I walked into Dr. S's office, and understood that much of my life was no longer in my control. Propelled into an examination room and asked to strip to the waist for a photo shoot, my first thought was that I'd had no time to fix my makeup or comb my hair. Should my glasses remain on or not? I was so not ready and so not thinking.

Dumb me. These photographs were to be of my body, nude from my neck to my waist, detailing my breasts. With the camera's first click, the reconstruction process began. In a strained semi-silence, two strangers, a patient and her doctor, attempted to make the best of a dreadful series of events.

Dressed, I met with Dr. S in his private office. Spread before me were pictures of the breasts of women, all of whom had undergone life-defining bilateral mastectomies. Indiscriminate in shape and size, these breasts all bore the scars of surgery.

I wondered if these women were still alive or if these photos were all that remained of their physical selves. To think that my breasts might become the latest addition to this assemblage for review made me ill. I turned away.

The thought of my one, self-contained cancer cell becoming invasive had terrorized me for the past six months. It had now done the unthinkable, and I was to undergo a bilateral mastectomy in six weeks. Fresh lines would be carved into my breasts, scarring them permanently. Forever disfigured, they would act as a harsh and constant visual reminder of my past, my present, and the precariousness of my future.

My breasts had comforted my newborn son and been presented to the world in my first training bra. Sex delighted them; sensitive to touch, they'd taken pleasure in being caressed.

After my bilateral mastectomy, much of what had been mine to share and relish would be missing. All breast tissue would be removed, as well as my nipples. Sensations in both breasts could be eliminated entirely. I could only pray that the surgery and ensuing medications would render me cancer free.

There were many baffling questions, the answers to which no one could foresee. Would I have the emotional and physical reserve necessary to face these changes, or would I retreat within myself, devoid of all emotions other than an appalling sadness, unable to welcome a lover's embrace?

My life had become a hideous freak show. No matter how irrational, in my mind, I'd warped into a social pariah.

CHAPTER EIGHT

Choices

Connected through our love of New York's energy and its depth of choices, Marlo and I became good friends years earlier. At the time she was the vice-president of a global design company. With a surgically sharp eye for color and style, it was fun to be with her. She kept me on point as to the latest trends.

Single and straight, our combined boyfriend stories were amusing, as were our occasional double dates. Together, we'd enrolled in fencing lessons, gone to the movies, and attended wine tastings, theater productions, museums, and any event that seemed interesting.

On a sweltering summer day years ago, we'd decided to bike on Nantucket Island off the coast of Cape Cod, Massachusetts. Trying to create a welcome breeze, I'd pushed ahead but soon realized Marlo had not followed.

Circling back, I found her seated crossed legged on the ground with a badly cut knee and matted hair. Twisted within the spokes of the bicycle lying nearby was the blue sweater that had been wrapped around her waist earlier in the day.

Marlo looked up at me, shook the sand from her hair, freed the ruined sweater from the bike, and said, "Shopping will make this all so much better."

With great energy, we'd diligently saved our money and planned a tour of the Amalfi Coast during the summer of 2001. We'd researched and discussed hotels, drivers, and points of interest as we dreamed of great food and wine, beautiful scenery, shopping, and all those handsome, sexy Italian men. Until my diagnosis of invasive breast cancer, all was "ready, set, go."

Not wanting to disappoint Marlo or myself, I evaluated my choices. I could undergo my scheduled lumpectomies, and then take to my bed to wait for my bilateral mastectomy. But as so many of my friends and family were already nervous because of my illness, I was determined not to surrender to my own anxieties. The best option for me was to have my lumpectomies and get out of Dodge. Italy would be cathartic.

I was well aware that most women facing breast cancer didn't have the luxury of a trip to Italy as a diversion, but for me to remain at home would have been of little value. The trip would help rebuild my spent physical resources as I geared up for surgery.

Having opted to reconstruct my bosom after surgery and open to changing my cup size and shape, where better could I research this subject than at an Italian seaside resort, resplendent with bosoms of every size and shape?

With her discerning eye, my good friend Marlo would help me decide which silhouette suited me best.

I called Marlo to tell her not only of my impending surgeries but also of my determination to follow through with our trip. I explained that by returning home just one day earlier than we'd planned, I'd be back in time for pre-op and ready to undergo surgery the day after.

That night, we met in the West Village to update our itinerary. As usual, Marlo looked great. Slim, blond, and blue-eyed with fine bones, Marlo never failed to present herself as fashion current.

Worried about my health and not knowing quite what to do, she offered me a cigarette from her pack of Galouises. Startled, I refused her and laughed. "Do you want to kill me quick? I already have cancer."

Mortified, she threw the cigarettes to the ground and said, "Oh my God."

We found a charming Italian restaurant and ordered a delicious meal with wine. Somewhere between our baked clams and mozzarella, tomato, pesto salads, Marlo leaned forward in her chair and asked, "Marge, are you sure you want to go ahead with your surgery? Why not have the lumpectomies and radiation instead and wait to see what happens?"

Reflexively, my body stiffened as I folded my arms across my chest to guard me from her next questions.

After a generous sip of wine, she put down her glass and continued. "I cannot believe that you've made this decision so quickly. Are you sure it's the right step to take?"

Bound to my chair by invisible ropes, I felt her words bore directly into my brain. Her questions were valid and deserved to be answered, but verbalizing my feelings about my breast cancer was hard to do. Each discussion made me feel pushed further into a corner.

After adjusting the scarf at her neck, Marlo said, "You're approaching this as if it were a project, something separate and apart from you. Are you really all right?"

I took a deep breath. My breast cancer had hit Marlo hard, and I understood her misgivings. She and I processed information differently and had contrasting styles of making decisions. Meticulous in her search for answers, she often sought a second and third opinion before coming to a conclusion. Though disciplined to get my facts straight, I generally followed my intuition above all else and sprung to action more freely. Nonetheless, digesting her words that evening was not easy.

I looked around the restaurant, trying to find a way to articulate my feelings.

"Look what I've done to you; this is awful," I started. I brushed my hair away from my face and went on.

"My body is breaking down in small increments. Between having a hysterectomy last summer and breast cancer now, I must abide by my intuition, as well as the medical information I've been given. For me to wait to find out if a course of radiation therapy is successful would be interminable."

It felt good to get it out.

"But if you don't take a breath and mourn this in some way…" Marlo's voice drifted for a moment.

"You are correct," I said. "Fighting cancer has become my project, otherwise I would break down, disintegrate, and disappear."

Marlo leaned forward, both elbows on the table, and whispered, her voice breaking from emotion, "We're best friends, and you've never shed a tear over this around me."

"I do cry, but only at home, and usually before I fall asleep, if sleep comes at all. To see my loved ones react to my unsteadiness just destroys me. Telling Matthew that I had cancer made me ill," I said.

Marlo sat back in her chair and listened. Once the door was open, I couldn't stop talking. "Matthew was fourteen when his father died of a heart attack. The possibility of his losing his mother would be a cruel blow to him." I took a deep breath and moved forward in my chair.

"Marlo, when we were little, our parents cautioned us to wear boots, zip our jackets, take off wet bathing suits, look before you cross the street, don't talk to strangers, and never, ever open the door when we were home alone. They never told us that we might get breast cancer or develop Multiple Sclerosis, Alzheimer's, or have a stroke. They hardly spoke of illness, and the details of death were mostly half-truths, alluded to in hushed voices."

Marlo raised her hand for a chance to speak, but my words filled the space instead. "For me to ruminate on why I developed breast cancer would be useless. Honestly, Marlo, why not me?"

CHAPTER NINE

The Assignment

Creating a bosom different from what I'd had before was something for me to consider, and the decision was mine alone to make. It was not open to debate or analysis and remained one of the few things I could control.

It would require research beyond what Marlo and I could accomplish in Italy. I needed a male perspective other than my doctor's, an evaluation predicated on more than clinical studies. Mutt would be the perfect addition to my small team of investigators. He'd dated and bedded almost all of the eligible women in New York City. Mutt's evaluation of which breasts held the most visual appeal would be valuable, plus his knowledge about which breasts, saline or silicone, felt best.

Since I had shared news of my invasive breast cancer with Mutt, not a day passed without us communicating. Sitting side by side, our delight in each other was obvious; one could naturally presuppose us to be lovers.

We were not.

With his encouragement, I'd taken control over that which I could. Accepting that I would never be able to go back in time to when I didn't have cancer, nor would my breasts ever again be what they once were, it was best for me to move forward.

Just days before I left for Italy, I found him at a bistro tucked away in a crease of New York City's real estate. With his back against a brick wall, he reigned over an imaginary court. He was dressed in tailored dungarees with a cobalt blue cashmere sweater tied around his shoulders over a long-sleeved black tee. Short and pudgy, Mutt was not conventionally handsome, but wrapped in flawless olive skin and topped with a mane of silver hair, he was most appealing.

I entered the room and felt his eyes caress me. We ordered drinks, a gin martini for me, and club soda for him. His non-alcoholic choice still caught me off guard. For many years, Mutt had closed down the best jazz joints in the city. Each night the bartenders had bundled him into a cab so that he was safe until the next night. Now fighting a heart in disrepair, he'd quit drinking alcohol without looking back.

After nibbling on some empanadas, I put my fork down and moved near enough to him that our arms touched.

"Mutt, I need your help." His head whipped around to face me. I had his full attention.

"Breasts come in every shape and size. In order for me to decide which would be right for me, I need your input."

Uncharacteristically, this man of many words said nothing.

"Should my implants be filled with saline or silicone? Between the two, which would look and feel the best?"

His dark eyes opened still further as I continued, "During my two weeks in Italy, you must conduct a very detailed, hands-on study, and report your findings back to me."

Laughter bubbled up from his toes before exploding through his mouth. After catching his breath, Mutt agreed to my request. "It would be my pleasure to serve you," he said, promising not to rest until he'd amassed sufficient data.

Then he draped his arm firmly around my shoulder, brushed his lips next to my ear, and whispered, "Remember our promise to become lovers before either one of us died?"

I nodded yes, impatient to hear how he would express his unending request to bed me.

"Just in case something does happen to you, don't you think we should move things along and sleep with each other now? Just think, I'll have a tender, sweet memory to sustain me through my years of missing you."

A swift kick to his shin was my answer. As he doubled up with feigned pain, I said, "Let's get out of here and take a walk."

We ambled along Mott Street, enjoying almost summer-perfect weather, as a warm breeze tapped lightly on the back of my neck. Mid-block, a shapely, middle-aged woman walked toward us wearing a form fitting red jersey dress.

As soon as she'd passed us, Mutt rotated on his heel to follow her. Intrigued, I stopped and turned around to watch Mutt in heat and on the prowl.

With little effort, he skillfully leaned into her personal space and spoke to her. She smiled, nodded, and stopped walking to throw back her shoulders and laugh. He continued to talk as she moved closer to him and accepted his proffered card. Then he gestured to me.

Within seconds she lifted her gloved hand, slapped Mutt hard across his face, tore his card in half, and walked away. As she stormed off, she screamed, "Disgusting!"

Mutt was usually so smooth. A charmer on command, he was always respectful of women. Whatever could he have said to infuriate her?

"What just happened? What did you say to her?"

"Nothing. I did nothing but tell her she was a spectacular woman."

"I guess she must have an issue with accepting compliments. Is that why she slugged you?"

A sly smile began to inch across his face. Ever mischievous and playful, Mutt bordered on evil, but it was a good evil.

"Well, that's not all I said."

"Yes, there's got to be more."

His smile expanded still wider as he continued. "I said that I'd love to have drinks with her sometime and if she were available, to please call me. Then I gave her my card."

"Okay..."

"Well," he continued, "I pointed to you and told her that you were my sister and that you were very sick and needed to have your breasts redone shortly and, as you thought hers were great, you'd sent me to find out if they were real or not."

"Oh Mutt, beyond not smooth. Did you want to date her or check out her breasts?"

"In all seriousness," he replied, "breasts were my primary focus. A date would be just a bonus."

I couldn't help but laugh. "Mutt, if you want to survive your interviews, I think you'd better tone it down or be more direct after a drink or two."

I kissed his reddened cheek, took his arm, and continued down the street.

Ladies, if in fact, during a two-week period in July 2001, an impeccably dressed stranger invited you to participate in this study, and you agreed to do so, I am most grateful for your contribution.

CHAPTER TEN

Italy

Still tender from my most recent lumpectomies and eager to run from the insanity of my anticipated surgeries, Marlo and I boarded the plane for Italy, hoping my anxieties would choose a different flight.

To my dismay, my anxieties were waiting in the terminal when Marlo and I landed in Naples. An unruly bunch, these worries rudely shoved each other while waving frantically at me. One looked like a surgeon and twirled a scalpel between his fingers. Another wore a nurse's uniform and held a huge hypodermic needle as if it were a dart aimed at my bosom. A disgusting figure dressed in rags dragged an empty coffin behind him. Two more juggled pink balls between them. Looking more closely, I realized they were flinging my breasts.

Horrified and angry, I turned to Marlo and said, "I need a drink. Let's find our car and get out of here."

As she went to find our driver, I spun back to face my unwanted travel mates, frustrated that I would have no respite from them.

Motionless, they looked at me directly and began to fade away. But my head felt like they'd placed a clock inside my brain that was counting down the days until I returned home to undergo my surgeries.

Before I could sink into despair, Marlo pulled up in our car and said, "Hop in. We have a long ride before we can get that drink."

I put the luggage in the car's trunk, slammed it shut, got into the car, and leaned back in my seat, hoping to get through the next two weeks without too much anguish.

In less than an hour, we'd reached our destination. Marlo and I were a mess. Although hot and weary, I insisted we go to the hotel's rooftop bar for a drink.

With visible reluctance, Marlo followed slowly behind me, lamenting, "I'm a tired, sweaty, wreck. I hate Italy. I want to go home."

Gently, I took her arm and propelled her up to the top of a grand staircase, through a massive archway, and onto a landscaped patio. Spread before us was a breathtaking view of the Amalfi coast.

Thrilled by its beauty, we hugged each other and laughed. Then we sat down at a small table and ordered a martini for me and a glass of Pinot Grigio for Marlo.

As we waited for our drinks to arrive, I asked Marlo, "Do you still want to go home?"

She smiled, brushed her hair away from her face, and replied, "Are you crazy? I never said that. I'm never, ever going home."

Once we had our drinks in hand, we tapped our glasses together and whispered, "To us." We remained on the patio long enough to watch the sun go down and finish another round of drinks.

After sundown, we bathed and rested, and then we went downstairs to our hotel's outdoor restaurant. There, we ordered some local wine, both red and white, and followed the waiter's suggestion to try the restaurant's tasting menu, which highlighted the region's fresh vegetables and pastas. It proved a great choice.

From our table, we could see the lights of the village turn on one by one. I imagined a band of fairies had lifted their delicate wands upward and now danced delicately to music only they could hear.

Gradually at first, then with increasing speed, the gentle specks of light ran together, and my morbid speculation returned as they transmuted into the brutally bright, invasive lights of an operating room. I gulped from the large glass of wine set before me, picked up my fork and began to eat, hoping to swallow the image.

"Marjorie, what is wrong?" Marlo questioned.

I hesitated but couldn't turn away without an answer. "In two weeks, I will never be as I am now."

Once we paid the check, Marlo pushed her chair away from the table and said, "Come with me."

As we made our way along a winding stone path, we passed shops still open. I tried to stop at one store, but

Marlo pulled me away and said softly, "Shopping must wait until another day."

She climbed higher up the narrowing path until we reached its end. In front of us were the damaged steps of the village church, which we'd passed earlier in the day.

Following Marlo into the recess of the worn building, I sat down next to her in an ancient pew. Nodding to me she said, "Let's close our eyes to pray for your good health."

With bowed head, I prayed first for those closest to me, and reminded myself that I had been blessed with their presence in my life. My health was an accident of birth, no more no less, but before I lifted my head and opened my eyes again, I turned my prayers inward to my soul and asked God to help me stand straight and tall and not burden those I loved with my fears. Then, I moved closer to Marlo, and held her hand until twenty minutes later she'd finished her prayers.

Afterward, Marlo and I returned to the hotel to sleep. As my eyes began to close, I remembered the assignment I had given Mutt before leaving for Italy. I chuckled at the thought of him approaching women and asking them personal questions about their bosoms, but if anyone could manage that, it was he. Nonetheless, it was prudent for me to get cracking and do my own research.

This task was made far easier by the fact that, after having spent our mornings apart, Marlo and I met each day for lunch on the beach. She and I had different body rhythms. She slept late. I was awake before dawn. She enjoyed reading in a chair on the beach. I enjoyed reading by the pool. She lingered in shops. I was quick to make my purchases and leave. Both of us needed time alone.

Our table always faced the beach, which though not having been designated as being topless, it most definitely did support the nearly nude display of women's breasts.

I was alert to them all.

Some were round, some oval, some tear-dropped, worn with varying degrees of bravado. Some were hidden beneath shirts, others dangled precariously over the tops of bathing suits. They were jaunty, perky, or flat; some seemed sadly neglected or depressed.

At every meal, I would prod Marlo: "How about those breasts? Do you think them too small, too large, too round, or not?"

Not long into lunch on the third day of this, Marlo put down her utensils, exasperated, and spat out, "Marjorie, you're making me crazy. I can't enjoy my meal while trying to answer your questions."

Textbook Marlo, I thought. I stayed quiet as she took another bite of pasta.

After she swallowed, she said, "Okay, my dear, I have a plan."

She asked for a pen and paper, and in no time, she'd devised a rating system by which to evaluate any bosoms I deemed worthy. Judged on a scale of 1 through 10, only those breasts praiseworthy of a 9.5 or higher would be included on the list.

Consideration was given not only to the size and shape but also to how well they would integrate into my body type. This means of classification kept me focused on my task and permitted Marlo to eat in peace.

In two weeks, I'd gathered enough information to use as a basis for my breasts' reconstruction.

When Marlo sensed my spirits flag, she would find a church in any town we visited and guide me there to pray until I, too, became a willing pilgrim who welcomed the calm and felt closer to God.

Although my vacation was tempered by an ever-present sadness, I'd been blessed to enjoy rich moments supported by a patient and caring companion. Though I believe faith transcends the body, and prayer can be given up any time, for me to have sat next to Marlo in silent devotion had been a tremendous comfort, and better prepared me to face my surgery when my clock ran out.

CHAPTER ELEVEN

August 1, 2001
Pre-Op

Having left Italy the day before, I was back in New York and jet lagged, but even so, I made an anxious dash to the hospital for pre-op tests. Scheduled for surgery the next day, I felt backed into a corner, hot-wired to blow, but with no time to explode. I rushed back to Brooklyn with a mental list of important must-dos: hair, fingernails, feet, and buy some food.

My colorist of more than twenty years, Gina, had coordinated all my salon treatments, which allowed me to waste not a moment. She'd surely correct my hair, damaged by the fierce Mediterranean sun. She would re-dye it a deep, rich auburn, threaded with copper highlights. As the colorant set, my manicurist would restore my fingernails and feet.

I couldn't control what was happening to me internally, but damned if I wasn't going to try to control the external.

To look my best under these lousy circumstances would be a tonic.

Gina and I locked eyes immediately as I walked into the salon. Motioning me to her chair, she said, "Sit down." In an instant, she whipped a leopard smock around my shoulders with the speed and ease of a magician. After tying it loosely under my chin, she ran her fingers through my hair.

"What a mess," she sighed. "It's faded and dry. You managed to kill off my masterpiece in ten days."

Pleased with her evaluation, she bent close to me until no one but me could hear her say, "Not to worry, when I get finished, you'll be the best looking patient in the hospital." As she breathed too deeply and wiped a tear from her eye, she kissed my check and added, "I so hate that this is happening to you."

I looked through my glasses at her reflection in the mirror. Full figured, fair skinned, blond, and appealing, her well-intentioned behavior demoralized me.

"Please, please, Gina," I whispered, "don't go there. If you fall apart, I will never get up from my chair."

Nodding yes, Gina squared her fleshy shoulders, kissed me again, and left to conjure up her secret mix of colors.

As I waited for her to return with her magic concoction, I remembered that patients needed to have one fingernail left without polish so that during surgery the technicians could monitor the flow of blood to the far reaches of their bodies. If the nail turned blue, the patient was in distress. With all the machines and specialists monitoring me, I could only hope that something or someone would notice my difficulty before waiting to see if a nail turned blue.

A little more than three hours later, I was finished with my spa services. With beautiful hair, well-pedicured feet, and perfectly manicured fingers, nine of which were painted a bright shade of coral, I was impatient to be done with my list of must-dos.

I paid my bill and went to Gina's station to give her a well-deserved tip, but before I reached her she intercepted me and managed to move me outside, beyond the eyes and ears of the salon's staff and clients.

Flamboyant in every way, she was dressed in New York City basic: a flowing, knee-length tunic and tights, both black, each covered with an abundance of multicolored rhinestones, so she looked like exploding firecrackers. She pulled me close against her generous body and said, "Tomorrow, I will go to church to light a candle and pray for your good health."

Other than familial and obligatory baptisms, births, weddings, and funerals, Gina could not be considered a regular communicant. Preferring to communicate with God on her own terms, her voluntary visit to church to make such a public display of faith was huge.

I hugged her without words, deeply touched by her sincerity, and then backed away to my car.

Although my short list of must-dos was almost complete, I still needed to buy food. Tomatoes, carrots, lemons, apples, peaches, and plums made their way into the shopping basket. Adding a jar of raspberry jelly and rye crackers, it was time to go home.

After parking in the garage, it hit me that it would be weeks before I could use my car again. My independence was solidly linked to my ability to drive. To let someone else take the wheel would be tough, but it was what it was. I hoped for patience.

With a sigh, I stepped down from my SUV and removed two small packages of food. I hesitated a minute before locking its door, as if to shorten the time of separation. After a minute or two, I shrugged my shoulders in resignation, clicked the doors shut, and went to my apartment.

I strode into my kitchen and saw packages of light blue paper cups, plates, and napkins strewn about its counter tops. Who made this mess?

It took a few moments for me to remember; I was the culprit of the disorder. I'd placed these items on my waist-high counters to avoid straining to reach for them in the over-my-head cabinets after I had surgery.

Detesting the idea of being homebound for even a few weeks, I'd splurged on expensive Italian bed linens. King sized, they were creamy white, edged with a light blue stripe, and soft against my skin. The sheets along with three lovely new nightgowns—milky white, gentle pink, and baby blue—were a soothing gift to myself that I hoped would help the healing process.

It was only nine o'clock in the evening, too early for bed, so I walked into the den to relax. Instead of turning on the television, I answered the first of many calls from one friend, two friends, three friends, and four more, each nervous, wishing me well, and asking if they could help before or after my operation. Other than suggesting that they have the surgery for me, I said their prayers would do quite well.

The phone finally stilled well past ten o'clock, and it was time for me to reassure Matt and Jodi that I was fine. Whether they believed me was hard to tell, but for certain, they humored my good intentions.

Maxie was my last goodnight.

Her predictable lament was a comfort. "Remember that I need to pick you up at six o'clock tomorrow morning?"

"Yes, Maxie."

"You do know that is very early for me to be awake?"

"Yes, Maxie."

"Well, I must sleep, quick."

"Good night, Maxie."

The woman never failed to make me laugh or cry. At that moment, I chose to laugh.

CHAPTER TWELVE

Night

As I lay in bed trying to capture sleep, I remembered floating on a raft in the middle of Mutt's pool and was happy in the memory of the warmth of that summer day. I'd morphed into a vapor, no longer connected to anyone or anything, free to drift, forever content, and blissful in my ignorance that within months, I would be diagnosed with invasive breast cancer.

Tomorrow, I would undergo a bilateral mastectomy. Touching my breasts, I found it difficult to believe that the tissue inside them could kill me, but the reality lay within my hands. Desperate to obliterate my thoughts for what remained of the night, I turned off the phone, downed a sleeping pill, and closed my eyes.

CHAPTER THIRTEEN

August 2, 2001
Ambushed

Early the next morning, I woke wishing the day would pass without me. Sad beyond words, I'd tried to pretend that I was all right. There was no way for me to really prepare for what lay ahead other than with a silent prayer.

After bathing, I dressed in my favorite pink cotton pajamas. Leaving the top unbuttoned, I tied its ends at my waist over a white bandeau, pinned a silk gardenia to a lapel, and went downstairs to meet Matthew and Maxie, who were waiting in her car to take me to the hospital.

With a broken spirit, I entered the lobby of the hospital just as the morning's sunlight flooded through its towering windows and onto its cold marble floor. I felt as if I'd entered a modern cathedral and prayed not to be sacrificed on its altar this day.

I'd neglected to select a room for my hospital stay and needed to go to the fourteenth floor to do so at once.

Perhaps I'd hoped for a last minute cancellation of the day's program because quite logically, if there were no room, there would be no surgery, which in turn meant there was no cancer.

Unfortunately, I could not wish my cancer away.

As I exited the elevator onto the fourteenth floor with Maxie and Matt close behind me, I heard the creepy voice of the woman who, months ago, had called to tell me of my "good fortune" in having a treatable form of cancer. At that point, I'd sensed that her agenda had gone beyond good fellowship. She'd overwhelmed and depressed me. To be in such close proximity to her now was frightening, so to avoid any chance of being ambushed as we walked past each other in the hall, I spun to my right and let my antagonist pass me on the left.

After deflecting this near hit, I was immediately bushwhacked by a starched, unsmiling man wearing a depressing black suit. Introducing himself as the floor's "concierge," he began to describe the merits of each of the available rooms. It was bizarre. Perhaps I could get a massage in my room? How about a privately stocked mini-bar after my surgery?

It all seemed too silly. This was a hospital, not a spa. All I wanted to do was to go to sleep, wake up, and leave the hospital quickly, preferably cancer-free. To be rid of him, I chose the first cozy room I stumbled on and let Maxie and Matt attend to the details. After putting away my things, I turned to look at the empty bed that would soon become either my best friend or my worst enemy.

CHAPTER FOURTEEN

Curtain Up

In a sterile pre-op suite, I met Dr. S. Standing uncovered in front of him the second time was not all that shocking. Today, in place of a camera, he held a broad black marker. By drawing thick lines up, down, and across my bosom, he created a lively blueprint for surgery on my exposed flesh. When finished, he instructed the nurses to prep me.

When I felt the pressure of a gentle but insistent pull on my arm, I understood that the curtain would soon lift, and I would be at center stage, lying on a stretcher with an IV drip stuck into my vein. This was not a dress rehearsal but, quite literally, my opening number.

Wanting to retch, I bolted from the stretcher to the bathroom, startling the attendants. Wearing only a hospital gown, with a bold map charted over my breasts, a tube dangling from my arm, where oh where did they think I was going?

I was spared throwing up; however, as I relieved myself in the bathroom, I realized this was my final opportunity to say, "No, I'm not ready for this surgery. Take these tubes out of my arms, give me my clothes, and let me go home." This thought tempted me more than I wanted to admit, but the idea of not having the surgery scared me even more.

I left the bathroom and found two nurses standing on either side of its door. The taller one looked down at me and asked, "Marjorie, are you okay? Do you want to leave now?"

Looking at them both I answered, "I'm not okay, but I am going through with my surgery." Then, I turned and walked back to my waiting stretcher, where I crawled onto it and once again faced my son and his grandmother.

Nothing could be said that would erase the fear and sadness I saw reflected from their eyes. So we kissed and we hugged until the attendant pulled me away from them. I turned my head and looked back at the space I'd just filled, now empty. Trapped in the present, I had neither a past nor a future.

Blinded by painfully bright, unforgiving lights, I could barely make out the figures encircling me as I lay on the operating table. Their voices were ever so soft against the harsh scrape of metal instruments.

I was frightened. Though wrapped in two heated blankets, I was too cold. I wished to disappear and reappear in a quiet, gentle place surrounded by friends and family. My prayer was to survive the coming procedures and not become another anonymous statistic marking an unfortunate surgical death.

Six months earlier, I'd lain on a similar operating table, waiting for the first of my lumpectomies to be performed.

In a room adjacent to mine, a woman had been prepared for a mastectomy. I had prayed for her and hoped it would not be me.

Now it was my turn to pray for myself and to wonder if she'd been as frightened as I, resigned to her fate, yet wanting so much to live. Had moments of her life flashed through her mind? Did she think of her death or of the quality of her life should she survive surgery?

Was she afraid to ask for more than a minute, or did she realize that to focus on what lay before her might devastate her completely? Did her heart break when she said goodbye to her loved ones? Did she finally cave in from the force of an incessant stream of terrifyingly bad news, which placed us both on operating tables, fighting for our lives?

At that moment, my death was as real to me as my life. I had invasive breast cancer, and as soon as I fell asleep, strangers would cut my body open to perform a bilateral mastectomy.

Something was injected into my IV that set my arm on fire.

I struggled to get up from the table, but my body no longer responded.

I must get away now, I thought, or they will have me for sure.

I am stone.

I belong to them.

CHAPTER FIFTEEN

Recovery Room

My chest felt as if an army of forks had gouged its tissue out piece by piece. Panicked but impotent to defend myself, I believed I had died and been damned to hell.

Hearing my son's voice and then feeling the pressure from his careful kiss on my cheek reassured me that I was alive and in the recovery room. Desperate to comfort him, I struggled to speak but could not. Smothered by pain, I blacked out.

Later that evening, I woke in agony. My medication was either wearing thin or not strong enough. I needed relief and tried to call for help, but too weak to be successful, my voice was but a breath of air.

Standing beside my bed, my son. Alongside him was my nurse Anne. Understanding my struggle, she asked me if I needed pain medication, nodded yes to her own question, and left the room.

Wearing a weary smile, Matthew looked down at me and said, "Mom, I know you feel like you fell on a land mine, but you are doing just fine. Hang on; the nurse will be back in a minute."

Looking down at my minimally but tightly bandaged breasts, I could see no obvious difference other than some marginal swelling. Into both of them had been placed drains: long, thin rubber tubes with peculiar, textured things shaped like grenades attached to each end. My parallel was fitting, for I'd surely gone to war, been blown apart, and had the insides of my breasts dug out like melon pulp.

Anne returned with a long syringe filled with my medication. As she emptied the liquid into my body, I felt a warm, comforting rush of relief. If this was the high a junkie craved, get out of my way and sign me up—it felt that damned good.

Incredibly hot, my body welcomed the bed's cool sheets against my skin, but I was stifled by my surgical gown and wanted it removed fast. As Anne helped me strip down to bandages and some generic bottoms, I whispered to Matthew that he should pretend I was wearing a bikini top and we were just sunning ourselves on a pristine beach.

To endure surgery, reconstruction, and then a lifetime faced with the uncertainty of a recurrence of cancer was problematic, but to have my child witness my ordeal was far more wretched. He deserved better. He deserved a healthy mother, not one in a hospital bed. Only when I'd fallen into a troubled sleep hours later did Matthew leave Anne to care for me throughout the remainder of that long, hard first night.

Having lost all sense of time, I drifted in and out of consciousness. At one point I saw a large, round head barely brush against the ceiling and then move quickly downward. Just before it crushed me, I screamed.

Anne jumped up from the chair and turned on the overhead light. The quiet "night monster" was an oversized, happy-faced balloon anchored to one of my flower baskets. Anne and I laughed, but I was so shaken that I needed medication to calm my nerves.

Later, Anne handed me a note and told me that Jodi, my daughter-in-law, had checked in on me at three o'clock that morning. Jodi was a labor and delivery nurse and worked on the tenth floor of the same hospital. Unable to focus, I asked Anne to read it.

"I'm watching over you. Love, Jodi."

I whispered, "I love you, too," and kissed the front of her card. Then I fell back to sleep.

Drains, pain, fear—that first night after surgery was very difficult. Anne helped get me up from the bed and go to the bathroom. Seated on a low stool, she emptied my drains by running her fingers along each tube, pushing my body's fluid down into the oval containers. When the containers were full, she detached them and squeezed the murky liquid out into the sink. I watched part of me spiral down the drain and prayed that what remained would be cancer-free.

After she'd reattached the ends of the drains, she gently sponged my tired, sore body with soap and words of encouragement. I was weak, and she was strong. I had no voice; she offered me her own. For the moment I was safe and grateful to have survived.

Early the next morning, Anne was relieved for the day by Moira. Standing barely five feet tall, Moira was definitely a leprechaun disguised as a nurse. With great care she helped me bathe, brush my hair, and apply some makeup before she deemed me ready to leave my room for a stroll down the hall.

One of my arms rested on top of Moira's shoulder, the other pushed my IV. My modest yet monumental goal was to walk down the length of the corridor twice, but Moira insisted we do four. We did four. I was exhausted and wanted to sleep, but Moira insisted that I eat. I refused, but wee Moira triumphed and cajoled me to do so. Lucky for me, Moira always won.

The second night after my surgery was kinder than the first and less dramatic. The pain had converted to a chronic, sharp, gnawing ache. I found my voice and ate a bit more than before. Sleep became easier, but that was due to exhaustion and drugs rather than emotional release.

The next morning, Moira helped prepare me for some company. Having experienced my share of post surgical spit up, I pulled together something to wear from a cart of clean, but generic, hospital gowns.

Elegant in its simplicity, my first layer fell to my knees with a not-too-subtle opening in the back. Too revealing and way too chilly, I closed the drafty gap by reverse draping a gown identical to the first over my shoulders.

I set off with Moira's help to find the fourteenth floor's lounge but stopped first to look in a mirror, to see what others saw when they looked at me. It was not at all pretty.

Bent at the waist, I moved like a snail. Though my hair was combed and blush was brushed onto my cheeks, strain stubbornly clung to my face. Only semi-mobile, I looked like a hag who, at best, was barely alive. Fixing a smile on my face, I stepped into the visitors' room.

With my entry, the group's energy visibly dimmed. It was an ill-disguised signal of concern for me, rather than any inhibition in their conversation. Inside the cheery yellow room, Marlo and Ava were nestled together on one of the room's two flowered sofas.

Predictably, Maxie sat alone in the one large, winged chair.

It was good to see them all, especially Ava, whom I'd spoken to but not seen since my return from Italy. I'd been busy with pre-op and she with her baby. I walked to her first and let her take me in her arms. Tears streamed down her cheeks as she held me as close as she dared.

"Oh Ava," I managed to say, "I'm going to be all right. The worst is over."

Calmed only a bit, she sat down, dabbed her eyes, and pulled herself together so that she could look at me with a faint smile on her face.

I sat down across from them all, Maxie, Ava, and Marlo, and remembered their prayers and how they'd fed my soul with encouragement.

"Where did you get that awful outfit? I could have brought you something else," Maxie said in great form.

Smiling, I fingered my gown and said, "You can each have something similar, just go to the laundry wagon outside, help yourselves. It's one size fits all, and better still, each is the same shade of blue. Make it your own by accessorizing. Marlo can help you."

No one moved on the idea.

These were bright, articulate women, but you wouldn't know it from their first attempts at post-surgery conversation.

"How is the food?" someone asked.

"Not too bad. I can order anything, but it's wasted on me. I have no appetite."

"Can you wash your hair?" Marlo asked before Ava added, "Are your nurses helpful?" I answered, "no" and "yes."

Understandably, these women were straining to make conversation, so I said, "Ladies, this small talk is making me ill. I'd feel so much better if you'd ask me anything you want to know."

Marlo was first. "Are you in a lot of pain?"

"Yes," I breathed.

"When do you start reconstruction?" whispered Ava.

"In about four weeks," I said.

"What can you wear? What can I buy you? Wraps and open shirts?" Maxie asked.

"Nothing, thank you. I will figure it out when I get home, though if you have an apron with side pockets, I can put the ends of my drains into them."

Ava asked, "Can you move your arms?"

"Yes, but not forward or back with ease. My chest muscles have been cut to accommodate tissue expanders, which will be filled with saline and stretched into my breast cavities. The worst of it is that I can't drive for a month."

This information stopped them cold. My car dependency was legendary. It took a moment for it to register, but after a gasp from each of them, Marlo and Ava volunteered to chauffeur me and take me out for airings.

Marlo's next question: "What's your prognosis?"

I lowered my head and said, "I can only hope for the best."

CHAPTER SIXTEEN

Step Together

Removed from the smells and noise of an oppressive August day, I could see a slice of Tenth Avenue directly from my window. Seated in my armchair, I watched as cars, trucks, taxis, and bicycles rudely edge each other for a sliver of space in which to move forward just a few inches.

Dressed in summery bright or New York City black, pedestrians walked deliberately down the street, guarding their personal space. Some clutched coffee containers close to their bodies as if they were trophies. A trio of elderly women scrambled to find refuge in a cleaning store to avoid being taken down by a horde of playful teenagers, as a homeless woman, layered with a heavy coat and sweater, defied the heat and pushed her broken cart down the street.

With predicable ordinariness, life on the avenue persisted, but emotionally parched and physically drained, I was insulated from its commonplace.

As I turned to get some water, I saw Dr. S standing at the doorway to my room. A kind and gentle man, he communicated intelligence and compassion.

Smiling broadly, he stepped toward me and said, "Hello."

Returning his greeting, I slid from the bed to prepare for his examination, but he shook his head no and said, "Today, I've come only to speak with you."

"Marjorie, you're doing well, and I believe that tomorrow you will be ready to leave the hospital to recuperate at home."

His words hit me with the force of a locomotive. Until that moment, I'd managed to avoid thinking about my life beyond my hospital stay. I denied nothing, but it had been far easier for me to stay in the moment.

For three grueling days, the hospital had sheltered me from the fragility of my life. Buried in its routines, it allowed me to remain on the periphery of my thoughts. Having compassionate strangers near at hand afforded me the freedom to feel as I wished without having to consider those closest to me. Emotionally raw, I was not ready to leave these buffers behind.

"I can't go home tomorrow. I'm weak, I'm tired, and I'm scared." Holding up my dangling drains for review, I groaned, "I still have these things attached to me."

Moving closer, the doctor took my hand and said softly, "I empathize with you and can only imagine how difficult it has been for you to undergo such challenging surgery, but you must trust my decision. I would not discharge you if I did not believe that you would do well at home."

Looking down at my drains, he said, "Later this week, I will see you in my office and remove these new best friends of yours. You will be just fine."

Ever so slightly I nodded my head in agreement, even though I still didn't believe I could manage anything.

After he left, I lay down on the bed, curled into a ball, and cried until Moira returned. Sitting down next to me, she put one of her arms across my shoulders and spoke to me softly. "In time, you will find the strength to rebound, but first, you need to cleanse yourself of all the anguish you've experienced these past six months."

Lifting my head, I looked at Moira and said, "Will I ever feel safe again? Will I ever trust my body and believe that I may have more than just a minute to live?"

"My dear, you've been traumatized mentally and physically. You are exhausted from the many changes you've made."

Taking my hand, she continued. "At times, life is just so hard to digest that it consumes all our strength and confidence. Patterns are no longer set, and comfort is constantly disturbed. In time, you will move forward, but right now, just curl up, let me order some hot tea, and give yourself to this moment where you at least have the opportunity to live."

Her words helped me put my life into perspective. I was lucky to be going home rather than be carried out, dead on a gurney, but I was down to my last nerve, shocked into the reality of my own impermanence. My resources had been sucked dry as I struggled to put one foot in front of the other since my initial diagnosis of cancer.

Going home tomorrow would be yet another test of my resilience because I would be prey to my own self-doubts. So be it. Life would just unfold as it would. I had little control except to show up and be counted.

I asked Moira for a sleeping pill, wishing to sleep through the coming weeks but settling for a few hours before my departure home. Second best would be good enough.

CHAPTER SEVENTEEN

Caravan

On the morning of my unwelcome departure from the hospital, I woke long before breakfast was served, still distressed and depressed. With unlimited arrogance, cancer had short-circuited my plan to move into Manhattan, retire from teaching, and start a to-be-decided next career. That plan was replaced with recovery, reconstruction, and ongoing visits with an oncologist.

The absence of long-range goals did not fit me well. Prior to my cancer, more often than not, I was energized, keen to explore and learn. At present, depression and apathy prevailed in my bone-tired body; to project past the now was difficult and upsetting.

As I began to get up from bed, something rubbed against my neck. Twisting my head to one side, I saw a lovely floral envelope slide down from the pillow. I reached inside and pulled out a matching card, signed by Moira and Anne.

Moira's signature jolted my memory, and I began to recall the essence of my conversation with her the night before. Essentially, she'd assigned me the responsibility for summoning my nerve to not only leave the hospital but also to put an end to this most discouraging period of diagnosis and surgeries.

Closing my eyes, I started to consider the pros of going home. I would regain my privacy and luxuriate in my own bed, safe in a sleep uninterrupted.

My garden would be a wonderful place for me to recoup my energy and reclaim my emotional equilibrium. To change my clothes at will and wear something other than a hospital gown of a color I now called "offending blue" could be added to my list of can-dos.

The heck with my drains—with two degrees, a Bachelor of Arts and a Masters in Education, I should be competent enough to pull these rabbits out of the hat. But then again, it was not unlike me to trip over the simplest of things.

"If there were sixteen ways to do something, Marjorie would find the seventeenth," was a valid assertion a friend frequently repeated. I could often complicate a straightforward solution by taking the most unnecessary and obscure steps to reach what should be a simple resolution.

After wiping my private tears from my cheeks, I started to dress in the same pair of pink pajamas I'd worn when admitted to the hospital. This time, however, the white bandeau would remain folded in my overnight bag. It was difficult enough to maneuver my drains, much less try to put on an elasticized top with no help from my severed chest muscles. With its buttons and deep pockets, the simple pajama top would be more than adequate.

Though it took me considerable time to pass my drains through each sleeve and put their end pieces into each side pocket without pulling them out, it was achieved. To raise my arms above my head was a challenge, so my hair remained uncombed.

A bit of powder on my too-pale cheeks and some mascara on my eyes made me look less ghostly; however, no one could mistake that I'd been on a vacation. Finished with my preparations, I was ready to leave, but waited for Maxie and Ava to help me home.

Though infuriated at my illness, Ava remained realistic to my needs and pushed her negative emotions aside to channel all her energy to bolster me. Direct, supportive and above all fair, Ava did not tolerate slackers at any level. Today, she'd twisted her schedule and left her young son with a babysitter so she could help me.

Ava was younger than I by almost fifteen years, but we shared equally, and often reversed, the roles of big and little sister. Our tight bond was centered on our honesty with each other, which at times could make us uncomfortable, but never failed to help us each grow.

Tall, blond, and attractive, her presence always registered, so when deliberate footsteps echoed down the hallway outside my room, I knew it was she. Wearing lightweight, long, blue shorts and a bright yellow shirt, she crossed into my room carrying a slew of empty shopping bags in which to put my things.

Dropping them on the chair, she put her arms tentatively around my shoulders, careful not to touch my chest. With tears in her eyes she said, "You made it. The rest will be hard, but the worst is behind you."

Quickly, I confided to her, "Maxie is hunting for bear and ready to explode."

Shaking her head with well-informed sympathy, Ava shrugged her shoulders and started to help me sort through the things I'd accumulated in the hospital.

We surveyed the room. Baskets filled with flowers were in varying degrees of fade. Attached to some were balloons, most of which had begun to deflate. Sent by friends and family, they'd initially cheered me, but now well past their prime, each signified something I no longer cared to dwell upon.

Without an appetite for the unopened, smartly wrapped boxes of candy, I relegated them to the nurses' station. A huge stuffed bear with a smart, pink "Fight Breast Cancer" ribbon tied around its neck was not something I would cuddle. Let a nurse take it home. Unused games and puzzles would go off to the lounge.

At some point I would respond to the many cards sent to me, so all of them would come home with me. Beyond that, I needed no tokens of my hospital stay. My wounded body would be keepsake enough.

Ava collected everything she could, filled the shopping bags, and left to redistribute them, closing the door behind her. Within seconds of her leaving, the door of my room flew open with such force that it crashed hard against the wall.

"If you still think that I am going to let you go home today and stay by yourself, you are crazy." Maxie stood in the doorway and caught her breath. "What the hell are you proving by staying alone? You have a family who loves you. Why are you being so selfish and not thinking of me?"

Deluged by her rant and too weak to summon either the energy or the will to pacify her, I braced myself for her next word wave to smack up against me and noticed how nicely Maxie had dressed for my attack.

That Maxie would at all times, dress well first and carry on second, no matter how real or imagined a crisis, always comforted me in its predictability. Spectacular today in her lavender Dior blouse and matching linen slacks, it amused me that I, dressed in lounge wear, was certainly her fashion antithesis.

A bundle of nervous energy and anxious well beyond her boiling point, Maxie continued to whirl and twirl about, making her long silk scarf dance behind her as if caught in a wind tunnel.

Turning to me, Maxie's flawless face became flushed, as her blue eyes narrowed. She spouted, "I just don't know why you put yourself and me through all of this? Why couldn't you have waited just a few more months and see what happened? Damn, you just had to do it your way. Can't you see that I am a nervous wreck, and I can't stand to see you suffer?"

I remained quiet. Despite having been present and privy to the most important conversations with my doctors, Maxie continued to be in denial as to the seriousness of my illness and disagreed with me on how I should fight my cancer.

Though I loved and respected her, whether she could move beyond her feelings was of no import to me. What did matter was for me to remain clear and comfortable with what my doctors and I believed to be my life-saving decision, which had been mine alone to make.

"Why the hell aren't you staying at my house? I just don't understand your thinking. You are just so damn..."

Stopping mid-sentence, Maxie switched her body around, alert to Ava walking back into the room.

Ever cool, Ava embraced Maxie, walked to my side and said, "Maxie, isn't it wonderful that the our girl has made it this far? It's great that she can finally go back to her own home." Ava's words had the unbelievable but wished-for effect of tempering Maxie.

After an uncommon moment of silence, Maxie looked back at me and calmly said, "I will get someone on staff to bring your release papers." Then she withdrew from the room.

Ava looked at my beaten face and said, "I wish I had gotten back here sooner, but everyone was so excited about the gifts we donated."

"It's fine, Ava," I sighed. "Maxie has been festering with these feelings for a long time. Most definitely, they will continue to rankle her for a bit more, but then again, as we both just witnessed, at least there is safety in numbers. Do you and the baby want to move in with me?"

At that improbable thought, she and I chuckled. Then she moved closer to me on the bed to wait for me to be officially sprung.

After signing my exit forms, first Ava, then Maxie left the room. Holding back for a moment, I looked at the bed one final time, thankful that for three life-defining days, it had welcomed me. I turned and walked out of the room on the fourteenth floor. Ready to be pushed into my future, I sat down in the waiting wheelchair.

CHAPTER EIGHTEEN

Return

Unlike the interminable elevator ride up to the fourteenth floor three days before, the ride back down to the hospital lobby was mercifully swift. It was there, on the morning of my surgery, I'd prayed not to die on the operating table. My appeal allowed Ava to now wheel me outside to Maxie's waiting car.

As she navigated me through the crowded expanse, Ava stooped close to me and whispered, "Marge, with your bosom bandaged, wrapped in tape and clear plastic, and with those drains hanging from each breast, you look like an unwanted Christmas gift."

I did look peculiar, but surrounded by the glut of midday workers scrambling to lunch, running errands, or trying to relax on their short breaks, it was easy for me to remain anonymous. None of them had the time or the interest to pay attention to a wan, middle-aged woman seated in a wheelchair wearing pink pajamas.

Outside at last, my first breath of air was anything but fresh. Mixed into the atmosphere were exhaust fumes, rotting waste, cheap perfumes, and dank body odors. It was a disagreeable cocktail, which caused me to gag.

Seeing my body round down, Ava jerked the wheelchair to a halt and rushed from behind to face me and shout nervously, "What's wrong? Are you all right? Should we find a doctor?"

I caught my breath, shook my head no, and said, "The stench here is just terrible."

"Welcome back to the Big Apple," was all she had time to say before Maxie commanded from the recess of her car, "Okay, girls, I haven't got all day."

Ava and I grinned at one other as she helped me curl into the back seat of the car. As she kissed me goodbye, she murmured, "Call me if you need anything at all." The car door closed, and within seconds, I felt Maxie's warm hand cover mine.

As the car moved along, I disengaged from the changing scenery outside my window and focused on my private thoughts. The preceding days had rendered me all but senseless. In the hospital, I'd left behind not only deadly breast tissue but also my innate sense of well-being. The future was unreliable at best, and mine seemed filled with far too many maybes.

Closing my eyes to rest, I fell into a brief, deep sleep and woke only when Maxie gently stroked my head and said, "Marge, you're almost home." Looking down, I saw that Maxie still held my hand.

Just as she and I arrived at my front door, Matthew opened it as if he had been standing on the other side; ready to spring to action at the first sound of me walking down the hall from the elevator.

With a tired but guarded smile, he stepped forward and wrapped his arm lightly across my shoulders, as if to apply any pressure would cause me to break.

Turning my head to him, I smiled and said, "Thank you for everything. I'm so sorry for causing you and Jodi so much concern."

Holding me a fraction tighter, he said, "Mom, not to worry, just rest. Why don't I stay with you tonight?"

"Matt, you and Maxie look awful, almost worse than me. You have circles under your eyes, and though she hasn't stopped eating from nerves, I think Maxie lost ten pounds. Remember, I slept through my surgery, you two did not."

Matthew shook his head and answered, "Mom, I know you need your space, but what happens if you're too weak to get up or if you feel sick in the middle of the night?"

Until now, Maxie had remained uncharacteristically quiet. However, Matthew's question became the perfect opportunity for her to jump in.

"You see, I told you the same thing. You can't stay by yourself. It's totally irresponsible. How can you manage by yourself? I will not let you and neither will Matthew. Haven't we worried enough?"

Satisfied to have finally vented her feelings, she stepped back, folded her arms across her chest, and turned to Matthew for support. She hoped I would cave in and either go home with her or let Matthew stay.

For me to hold my position took almost all of my strength. Their concerns were legitimate, but I was sinking fast and craved to be alone to catch my breath, at least for a few hours.

Choosing my words carefully, I said, "You're both right. I love you more than you will ever know, but just give me a little bit of time to process these past few days. We're all exhausted and need to rest. Tomorrow will come soon enough."

Matthew and Maxie looked at each other in defeat. They knew that no matter how irritating and irrational my logic, I would not change my mind. Matthew, followed by Maxie, kissed me goodbye.

They left, and I was relieved to be completely alone. Tired beyond the physical, my sole objective was to reach my bed, but when I saw my reflection in my full-length mirror, I stopped short.

Worn and thin, I looked like a kidnap victim whose ransom would be paid if only she still breathed. Curious as to what my remains looked like, I held my drains, removed my pants, and carefully maneuvered out of my shirt.

Spread over my body were scars, each a graphic reminder of a previous surgery. My hysterectomy had left me with a seven-inch horizontal line three inches above my pubic bone. Above that and to the right, a four-inch diagonal scar underscored a ruptured, gangrenous appendix, which had brought me close to death.

Another smaller scar, also diagonal, reaffirmed the seriousness of that episode, marking where a tube had been inserted to drain the toxins from my system. These scars were a road map of my life.

Added to these markers were those most recently etched firmly into my breasts. Though covered for the moment with surgical tape, they too would be everlasting tokens of my breast cancer.

The thought of what could happen to me still made me shudder. After having gone through so much, it still might not be enough to protect me from more cancer. I wondered where to find the strength to get up each day and not collapse back down from fear.

After putting on my bottoms again and reattaching the drains to my pants, I pulled myself onto my bed and sank down, down between my sheets and under my lightweight quilt. I was home at last.

One nod away from a deep sleep, the phone rang. Afraid of more bad news, my gut reaction was to not pick up the phone, but I figured it could be Maxie or Matthew; my money was on Maxie.

I was pleasantly surprised that it was the surgeon who'd performed the first part of my surgery. A remarkable woman, kept too busy with too many surgeries, she was nonetheless communicative and compassionate. She'd called to see if I was all right and to reassure me that truly believed my prognosis to be favorable. I thanked her for her call and said goodbye.

At this point, all that remained was for me to find peace within my life and to accept my body without viewing it as a betrayer of my trust. Too tired to take a sleeping pill, I closed my eyes and went to sleep. It was only six o'clock in the evening, but I felt like I'd been awake for a week.

At 11:30 the next morning, I woke and found myself still flat on my back, safe within the bunker of pillows I'd fashioned the night before. Intact and still secured to my pajama bottoms, my grenades. Many months would pass before I would again enjoy something close to a good night's sleep without alcohol or drugs.

CHAPTER NINETEEN

Reunion 1

Fortunately, my earliest days of recuperation were predictable, as the combination of general anesthesia and medications proved potent. For at least a week, my ability to think clearly or remember more than a minute was greatly diminished.

The pain in my chest was persistent and penetrating, but as each day passed, it receded into an annoying ache, which eventually faded away. As the nerves in my breasts had been cut during surgery and might never regenerate, the only sensation they now registered when touched was pressure.

Convalescing at home was a drill I knew too well. Each morning, I'd shower and try to straighten my bed, though it was not possible to do anything more than a show of tiny tidy. Dressing in something cool and easy boosted my spirits.

A wrap of cloth about my waist and a belly shirt or bikini top was fine, as each allowed movement without constriction while covering my bandages and holding my drains in place. Exhausted from these simple tasks, I'd nap and then try to read in my garden, but it would be no more than a page or two because, warmed by the mid-August sun and unable to concentrate, my eyes would quickly close.

Aware that this was my second major surgery in little more than a year, my friends and family kept their initial visits short, their telephone calls brief. However, convinced that I would starve to death, Maxie would not be deterred, stopping by each day with lunch.

Her visits were welcome, generous, and allowed us much-needed private time, though she never resisted an opportunity to chide me for not staying with her.

"Marjorie, you do realize how much easier it would be for me if you stayed with me and your father-in-law. Our maid and driver could help you navigate more easily."

I smiled as she recited her list of home-helpers, but she'd omitted the constant flow of people who habitually congregated at her home. Good food, fine drink, and, best of all, gossip was on the menu all day, almost every day.

"Maxie, all I can do is sleep and rest. Your house is a circus of people coming and going. The phone rings all the time. Staying there would just make me cranky and irritable."

She tossed back her head, laughed soundly, and grinned. Patting my hand she said, "You're so right, sometimes it overwhelms even me. Better still, during lunch, I'll just hide out with you."

"Agreed," I said.

When I was allowed to roam, I set out only as far as my body would allow. My chest's muscles were cut; lifting, carrying, and pushing were not to be considered. Because I could not drive, I felt much like a caged animal.

Undefined and vulnerable, frightened and gasping for air, I often felt as if I were crashing backward through space. I turned to my dear friend Mutt for solace, and he encouraged me to view these collapses as just temporary breakdowns of my spirit, points in time when I could reflect, regroup and restart my difficult journey. His advice prevented me from imploding, but it still remained for me to learn to live with the uncertainties of fighting cancer.

Though I'd called Mutt after my surgery, I couldn't bear to have him see me in the hospital and thought it might be a painful reminder of his own quintuple bypass. Now that I was home, I invited him to visit.

Between shifts at the hospital, Jodi stopped by and helped me get ready for my visit with Mutt. Stepping back for a final check, I realized that my breasts were fuller from having swelled after the operation.

Turning to Jodi I said, "Amazing, I've just undergone a bilateral mastectomy, and now I have a larger bosom than before."

Jodi chuckled and nodded her approval of my urban beach look. As she got ready to leave, she took my laundry, stuffed it in a backpack, and promised to return with it and Matthew the next day.

Before she left, the telephone rang; she picked up the receiver and handed it to me. The voice of my "cancer supporter" made me cringe.

"How are you doing?"

"Holding my own," I said.

Without hesitation and in a sarcastic tone, she shot back, "I guess you don't need to talk to me."

If possible, I would have reached through the phone and slapped her hard, but instead I mouthed the word "bitch" as I pointed to the receiver.

Repelled, I said, "Thank you and goodbye."

Would she have preferred me to be miserable, sobbing, climbing the walls, desperate for her support? She was supposed to be a light of hope and encouragement to women such as myself, not snarky and self-serving.

Soon after Jodi left, the doorbell rang. I looked up at the wall clock in the kitchen. Mutt was right on schedule.

As I opened the door with difficulty, Mutt stood before me, his arms filled with gardenias, my favorite flowers. Nodding a quick greeting, he walked into the kitchen, where he began to arrange the flowers in my vases. Following after him, I watched him focus on his task.

Finished, he faced me directly.

Looking first at my eyes, then down to my chest, then slowly back up to my eyes, he took my hands and led me to my bedroom.

Settling down across the pillows, he stroked the empty space next to him and reached for me. Wordlessly, he eased my way by holding the drains and gently laying me back onto the bed so that I faced him directly. Ever so lightly, he kissed my cheek. Safe in our friendship, I began to cry.

Mutt held me closer and murmured, "Baby Girl, I know how frightened and tired you are. It's difficult to face your own mortality. There never is a right time to do so.

"Nothing makes any sense at all, I know," he continued. "After my heart surgery, I was afraid of doing almost anything and wondered each day if this was the day I would die. In time, I was able to push those feelings behind a mental door."

"But," I said, "you're much stronger than I."

"Not so, but not speaking the words, I believed, would strangle my fears and make them disappear."

He kissed me again. "Your spirit will sustain you, and so will I."

I started to answer, but he put a finger on my lips, and said, "Quiet. Sleep, Baby Girl, sleep." Comforted by his words and physical presence, I finally did.

Within hours, I woke dripping sweat and painfully sore and dragged myself into the bathroom to sponge myself down. I didn't know what bothered me most, the drains, the perspiration, or the constant ache in my chest. Nothing felt good. I took some painkillers, left the bathroom, and started to go back into my bedroom.

Seeing Mutt sleeping peacefully across my bed gave me pause. In the morning, he would be gone. I would be sad, too eager to see him again and speak with him on the telephone. It was better for me to not allow myself to feel that close and connected, that needy. I went to the den to lie down on the couch and let the medications kick in.

During the night, I felt Mutt move beside me on the couch and lie down next to me on his side. Too tired to move, I kept my eyes closed, happy he'd followed me to the den. He kissed my head and said, " I love you, Baby Girl."

"I love you, too," I said before we fell back to sleep.

As daylight began to reveal the room, I began to move and felt Mutt still beside me. Without a word, his soft hands touched my cheek as he grazed my forehead with his lips before helping me up.

Smiling, he said, "I need to go, but will call you later."

Slowly, he opened the door and left, but not before turning to smile at me. Returning to my bed, I slept until the next round of pain and perspiration woke me again.

CHAPTER TWENTY

Gone Missing

I didn't enjoy the person I'd become and greatly missed the woman who was strong, well defined, and joyful. For me to harvest the will to accept that I faced a serious health issue was depressing. With limited control over my future, brief moments of calm were tempered by swells of alarm at the prospect of my death.

To share my concerns with friends and family was an option, but to present myself as being either lost or frightened rather than positive and strong would be a disservice to them.

Instead, I became proficient not only in verbalizing what I did not yet feel—"I'm just fine." "Yes. I slept well last night."—but also in redirecting conversations away from my health—"How are the kids?" "Where are you traveling to next?"

Miserable, I desperately needed objectivity and reached out to my former therapist, Ellen. Though she had retired, perhaps she'd agree to become a resource from which I might be able to secure clarity of thought and thereby emerge from my spiritual collapse.

I trusted her with my deepest emotions because we'd worked hard to slug through the issues of life, love, and death for at least four years.

After each visit with her, I'd feel as if I'd moved just a bit closer to developing the emotional tools needed to process and modify my behavior in order to become more positive and productive. Graduating from treatment had been my Nobel Prize for Self-Improvement.

Although we'd not spoken for at least three years, dialing the mix of seven digits plus one was instinctive. Recorded in Ellen's crisp, Philadelphian accent, her voice message had not changed and was a reassuring continuance of predictability.

Petite, poised, pretty, and well into her seventies, she'd always dressed in tailored suits during our sessions. Choosing colors that flattered her pale skin and light brown hair, she often seemed to be absorbed into the expanse of Central Park, which was visible behind her through the picture window in her office. I wondered if she'd kept the space?

At the sound of the beep, I exhaled quickly and blurted, "I need to speak with you as soon as is possible. I've crashed."

I resolved not to dwell on when she would return my call or whether she'd have the time to work with me again, and just as I realized I hadn't left my name or said hello in my message, the phone rang.

"Marjorie dear, what's wrong? Is Matthew all right?"

Knowing I valued my son above all else, Ellen's question was valid.

"Matt is fine," I reassured her, "but I was diagnosed with breast cancer in December and underwent a bilateral mastectomy one week ago. Ellen, I'm terrified."

"Oh my," she said gently. "How can I help you? I can only imagine what you've been through."

"Ellen," I sighed, "what the hell do I do?"

"Marjorie, I wish you'd reached out to me sooner, but just the same, we will work together and get you to a better place, I promise."

"Thank you," was all I could say.

We scheduled to speak at 1:45 the next afternoon. Ellen would be free, I would have napped twice, and Maxie would have come with my lunch, shared it, and left.

Maxie arrived the next day after my second nap. She unpacked the goodies she'd brought and said, "Marjorie, you look terrible. You're too thin, and I hate what you're wearing."

True, I was thin, but major surgery will do that to a person. My outfit of a wrapped cloth around my hips and a white, front-button shirt bored her. I responded with a shrug of my shoulders and smiled.

Although she frequently stretched my patience, it comforted me that she remained true to her character and loved to nit and pick. Perfection could only be achieved if one met her often obscure standards. It was not something I, or anyone one else, achieved with regularity.

Her visits often lasted little more than an hour, and by one o'clock she was usually gone. Today, she seemed to need to stay longer, as if to make sure that I was okay. She continued to gossip about this or that family matter as the time moved closer to 1:30.

I needed her out the door soon, or I would be late for my first session with my therapist. Not choosing to share this information with her because she might take it as a personal invasion of our relationship, I began to yawn, but she continued to chatter.

Finally, at 1:35, I stood up and said, "Maxie, I need you to go. I love you, but I'm just exhausted. She looked at me, shook her head and hissed, "You see, you should have stayed with me. You'd rest better, and I wouldn't need to make this trip to you every day. See you tomorrow. I love you."

With minutes to spare, I walked into my bedroom and watched the hands of the small clock on my night table move closer to 1:45. Our forty-five minute sessions had never started on the hour, always on the quarter to the hour.

As I waited for the phone to ring, I wondered what Ellen did during those fifteen minutes between each session. Perhaps she made a dash to the bathroom or drank a glass of tea from a delicate cup. Perhaps she took a power nap or transposed her mental notes to paper or computer?

The phone rang at 1:45, and soon after, I began to describe what had taken place during the past six months. Starting from the high of Matthew and Jodi's wedding, my narrative described my emotional slide onto my knees, which ended with me face down in mud.

"Ellen, I'm screwed. My life has become too sad and unpredictable."

"My dear, life is often just that, sad and depressing. What we can do is try to labor through it and gain some objectivity," she answered.

She reminded me that in order to cope, I often tried to minimize my feelings. She did not believe I was in denial, but felt that in order to be self-protective; I'd not yet fully absorbed how great the repercussions could be from this particular surgery.

"I don't understand," I countered. "I'm frightened, and all I want to do is stay in my bed and cry."

"Rather than accept your fears, you've always tried to move beyond them without first fully acknowledging them," Ellen calmly replied. "To spring back unscathed from these unfortunate experiences is difficult. It would be unhealthy to avoid the reality of the situation and would stifle your capacity to confront these feelings, work them through, and allow yourself to heal."

Counseling me to be patient, she reassured me that as I became physically and emotionally stronger, I would find myself again, though with additional concerns and sensitivities. To embrace my feelings, no matter how painful, would be a solid first step in letting them go.

Our conversation remained reassuring until she said, "Having had mastectomies, you need to accept the fact that your body has been violated, mutilated by your doctors."

My mind snapped to attention as these words pushed up against me hard. What the hell was she saying? Didn't she understand what I'd just shared with her? Only cancer had violated my body.

Tightening my grip on the receiver, I said, "Ellen, had I not undergone my mastectomies, cancer cells would have mutilated my body and ultimately killed me."

Panic grabbed me around my neck. My heart began to race. I stood up from my bed and paced the floor. Was I wrong to think that Ellen could help me?

As calm and controlled as ever, Ellen continued. "Are you experiencing some doubts about your self-worth as a complete woman?"

Her words stung me with the sharpness of an angry wasp, which caused my body to flinch in anger as I shot back, "I cannot believe what you're saying. What the hell are you talking about? Though badly bruised on many levels, I'm very much alive and do not feel as if my femininity or sexuality has been diminished. Though challenged by cancer, I do not question my completeness as a woman, but rather my ability to withstand the many challenges it presents."

Hardly above a whisper, she answered, "I understand how you feel." Then she asked, "Do you realize how passionate your response to me has been?"

My reply certainly had been animated. She was right. My passion had found its way home, but I was still uncomfortable with Ellen's questions.

I asked, "Did you really believe that I felt that cancer had mutilated me, and that I doubted my completeness as a woman? Did you manipulate me on purpose?"

There was silence on the other end of the phone, which made me uncomfortable. I was impatient to hear her response, but I remembered how she would often take long moments to process and respond to my questions or statements.

With measured words, she answered, "Marjorie, I needed to know how you really felt about your surgery. My questions were posed to help you frame your thoughts. Only when we both have a clear understanding of the issues involved can I begin to help you." She continued with, "You will need to relax into these exchanges without feeling threatened by any challenge to explain your thoughts. Our next session will be much easier."

Ellen and I agreed to speak formally each week, although she would be reachable during the times in between, which made me feel as if I'd been tenderly swathed in a plush blanket.

Having initiated this dialogue with my therapist, I'd become proactive in my psychological recovery. To make clear to myself that I'd never put my self-worth as a woman into the mix of considerations and that my need to survive took precedence over any attachment to my breasts as they were, "or the tissue within them" had allowed me to define my attitude about my surgery. It was a good start to rebuilding my spirit.

CHAPTER TWENTY-ONE

Drains

Within a week after surgery, I was scheduled to have my drains removed. Their departure would certainly be celebrated. Soon after my little pets were removed, I'd be permitted to shower and say goodbye to sponge baths.

Wanting to strike out on my own, I called for a car to ferry me to the plastic surgeon's office in Manhattan. Dressed casually in baby blue, cotton, waist-tie pants, I nodded a final thank you and goodbye to my drains before stuffing them inside my pants pockets for the last time. An oversized white-on-white striped man's button down shirt completed the look.

Slipping on some flip-flops, I was ready to go, but not before struggling to open my own front door. Having the car service driver standing outside with his car door open was a blessing.

Relaxing into the car's back seat, I marveled at the changes I'd undergone in less than a week. Without drains to tie me down, my mobility would be limited only by my body's recovery. Simple pleasures would now be possible, such as pullovers and things without pockets. Perhaps unfettered, sleep would arrive without as much struggle.

The day was sunny but carried the sense of autumn moving in quickly to chase summer away. If not too tired after my appointment, I would brave a stroll along Madison Avenue and window-shop at some of its elegant and expensive stores.

We arrived at my destination, a corner building on Park Avenue, on the Upper East Side of Manhattan. Unsolicited, the driver, a round, pleasant-faced man, extended his hand to help me lift up from the seat.

"Thank you," I said.

Smiling warmly at me, he said, "Feel better."

After I passed surveillance, the imposing door slowly swung open. I stepped down the three wide, marble steps directly into the suite of offices, which reminded of a beautiful boutique hotel rather than a surgeon's workplace.

Muted shades of apricot, the walls mixed well with the textured gray sofas and chairs. A pink-flecked, dark gray marble wall curved around the receptionists' bank of desks and computers. Floral arrangements positioned artfully along the divider gave it warmth.

Hidden behind French doors and beyond several examination rooms lay a fully equipped operating room, used solely for cosmetic procedures.

Delighted to see me up and about, though surprised that I'd come alone, the office staff stopped what they were doing and walked from behind their desks to greet me.

They surrounded me within seconds and congratulated me on having come through my surgery so well.

"Thank you very much," I said, as I kissed them on their cheeks. "Thank you for your support."

From the onset, the entire group of secretaries and nurses had been supportive and kind. Well trained, they'd coordinated every detail of my surgery, including pre-op tests, nurses in the hospital, which saved me from additional confusion and worry.

Initially preoccupied with my impending operation, I'd been somewhat removed and distant from their warmth and concern, but now, I could appreciate just how wonderful they were. Their energy gave me strength and encouragement.

Ushered inside an examination room, I was asked to remove my shirt and lay down on a table, with my drains still attached. Within minutes, the doctor was there to examine me. Carefully removing my bandages he said, "I'm so pleased; you are healing beautifully. Just relax and we will have these drains out in a flash."

Relax. That was the key to everything, but it was not yet part of my internal vocabulary, so I held my breath and anticipated the worst.

"Marjorie," the nurse said, "please breathe, it's important to your health." I started to laugh and did as instructed.

To minimize my discomfort, Dr. S. and his nurse positioned themselves on either side of my bosom. Each then took hold of the drain sticking out from the breast closest to them. After counting one, two, three, they simultaneously pulled out a drain. My pain was slight.

All that covered my incisions when I left was a thin, self-peeling strip of tape. At last I was free, but nonetheless exhausted from the ride to the doctor's office and the stress of the procedure. I opted not to window shop. Instead, I went home to shower...forever.

CHAPTER TWENTY-TWO

Oncologist

Sentinel nodes removed and tested at the time of my mastectomies indicated that, to insure my cancer would not spread, aggressive intervention was needed. One week after my drains were removed, I made my first visit to the head of Oncology at St. Luke's-Roosevelt Hospital Center, and I was scared.

To think my surgery might not have been enough to ensure my good health was daunting. Intellectually grasping the dynamics of the disease, I appreciated its unpredictable independence. One could be free from cancer one day but quite possibly on any day, month, or year thereafter, it could try to suffocate you again.

After signing my name on a generic registration sheet, I asked the guard to direct me to the oncology department. Just speaking the word unnerved me, as it remained too new to my vocabulary and was spoken with much internal angst when connecting it to myself.

Too uncompromising to be cavalier, cancer was something often whispered in hushed tones, as if to speak the word would bring it, free of charge, to your doorstep. Cancer was something other people struggled with, until it welcomed me into its arms with a life-extinguishing embrace.

It was alarming for me to now be standing in front of a door labeled Oncology as a patient, but to turn and run would deny me the opportunity of a rest of life. Gathering strength, I pushed the heavy door open and entered the hushed world of serious illness and proscribed treatments.

After registering, I shrunk into a soft leather seat and tried to disappear as a steady stream of patients walked past me down a long, long corridor. Some managed on their own, as others struggled with walkers. Those in wheelchairs needed caregivers to push them down the space.

Imaging myself slowly vanishing, I closed my eyes to this parade of sadness. Doing so did not make it go away, but gave me a visual respite from misery. Hearing my name called, I opened my eyes to see a tanned, blond, middle-aged woman. Dressed in a white lab coat, she held a clipboard in her hand and leaned against the reception counter.

As I rose from the safety of my seat and walked toward her, she smiled at me. Offering her hand, she introduced herself as Cindy, my oncological nurse practitioner.

With strong, deep blue eyes, she looked directly at me and said, "You'll be just fine. The doctor is brilliant."

Without my own history of success, I could not respond to her enthusiasm but managed a tempered nod yes.

Taking my hand, she indicated that it was my turn to walk down the long corridor as many had already done within the prior fifteen minutes. We walked until we reached a small room, which had two straight-backed black chairs located on either side of an examination table.

After sitting down in one of the chairs, she motioned for me to sit across from her in the other one. Now face-to-face, she proceeded to ask me what seemed to be a thousand questions regarding my medical history.

My answers sounded rote—"Yes, no, yes, yes and no, I do not know, check, check, check."

Despite my wariness, Cindy remained cheerful and kind. After having taken my blood pressure, she asked me to get on the scale. However, she did not insist.

As an adult, my weight had never changed more than a pound or two north or south of 116. Having thrown out my own scale years ago, I'd let the fit of my clothes be my guide. The connection between weight and cancer treatments had not yet registered with me, so I refused to get on the scale. There was so little I could control, I said no to getting on the scale, just because I could.

Within minutes, Cindy and I were finished with all of her preliminary chores and together left the room to meet with the doctor in his office. Passing the infusion suite, I was stunned to see patients, old and young, seated or laying down on massive recliners. Attached to each patient were snake-like tubes that drained cancer-fighting drugs into their arms from bags suspended above their heads.

This graphic depiction of cancer made me freeze in place until Cindy quietly led me away. As I moved away from these patients, all fighting so fiercely to live, I prayed for their health and hoped to never need to sit down, roll up my sleeve and join their ranks.

The oncologist walked from behind his large, cluttered desk to shake my hand. A pleasant, gray-haired, affable man in his late forties, he began to discuss with me my course of treatment as soon as I sat down in one of the office's three brown leather chairs.

Direct in his presentation, he believed that my having had a hysterectomy the previous summer was a good thing, as now I would be able to take my cancer therapy in the form of Arimidex, rather than undergo chemotherapy, without the risk of developing uterine cancer.

In addition, he would prescribe Effexor to control my outrageous full body sweats. These medications were strong and could produce an array of debilitating side effects, such as fatigue and body aches. These drugs would take as much as they gave, and would open a new chapter on my ability to cope, but it was worth a shot. With pre-scriptions held tightly in hand, I left his office and hoped for the best.

CHAPTER TWENTY-THREE

September 11, 2001
Back to Work

Slowly slipping into a post-operative depression, five weeks later, I returned to work too soon in order to keep what little remained of my sanity. Though my strategy was straightforward, I'd not only misjudged the level of my stamina, I'd forgotten that much of one's life is uncontrollable.

Believing that work would distract me from my personal hell, I was uncharacteristically eager to begin this particular school year. For five hours each day, my focus would be on something other than my health.

Throughout New York City, children and their parents separated from each other on the first day of school, September 10, 2001, with varied degrees of apprehension. Confident or not, the older children came to school on their own. The very young ones clutched their parents' hands; some laughed, cried, or fell into frightened silence, displaying no emotion whatsoever.

To step into a class line led by an unknown teacher was huge for the wee first-timers because it would tear them from the comfort of their parents and move them forward into a large and unimaginable classroom. I was one of those mysterious teachers.

On their first day of school, my class of multinational four-year-olds dressed to amaze, and amaze they certainly did. All the girls wore a best party dress, pants, skirt, or shirt, which were pleated, swirled, bubbled, straight, plaid, striped, or solid in every color combination imaginable. On each head of hair—straight, curled, wild, waved, or tame, blond, brown, black, or red—were colored bows, bands, or barrettes. They reminded me of animated life-size dolls.

Not to be upstaged, the boys turned out in pressed slacks or jeans topped with starched dress shirts or ironed casual tees, with their hair freshly cut and gelled to perfection. Barely holding onto some of their shirt collars were small clip-on ties. Picture perfect, the entire class was ready for a children's magazine shoot.

These Pre-Kindergarteners were precious, but for me it was never love at first sight. To trade the freedom of my summer vacation for the confinement of the classroom each September was difficult. But as the temperature cooled, and the leaves dried and changed their colors from green to red, yellow, orange, and brown, a love for my students would re-emerge. It was a predictable and lovely transition for me to experience each school year.

The next day, the children lined up with delight and moved more quickly to my classroom, where they hung up their sweaters and backpacks. After each washed and dried their hands, they moved to a low table to secure for themselves Styrofoam trays, plastic utensils, a small box of cereal, an individual carton of milk, and fruit.

Afterward, they carried their spoils to tables to sit down and eat. At this point my assistant, Juana, or I offered them an ever-changing hot component to their meals. Whether they ate was their choice, but it was our job to encourage them to try.

It was memorable to watch them thoughtfully make their own food selections and then participate in animated conversations, which detailed their favorite superheroes, pets, or movies. Children who were too shy to immediately join in these exchanges would usually jump into the mix later in the school year.

Minutes after 8:46, that morning, before the usual school-wide pledge of allegiance, our principal walked quickly into my room without her usual smile. A tall, slim, dynamic redhead, she looked more like a fashion model than an elementary school principal. Highly skilled, she'd elevated our school to a level of excellence in which its faculty, students, and parents took great pride.

Clearly troubled, she leaned to me and whispered, "A plane just crashed into the North Tower at the World Trade Center in lower Manhattan."

"Oh my God. How do you know?" I asked.

"I just received a relayed message from the Board of Education. We don't know how this will affect us yet," she answered.

Stunned, I looked at her and said, "Oh my God, this is awful."

She nodded and left to alert the rest of her staff.

Undoubtedly and unfortunately, both the pilot and his passengers had to have been killed; yet I believed it to be a fluke, a horrible mishap of modern day travel within the overcrowded skies above our city and gave little thought to the innate stability of the World Trade Center, whose Twin Towers rose high and city proud.

A vertical metropolis, it was composed of multiple companies, staffed by thousands, and thought to be invincible. After all, it had withstood the bombing of its underground public parking garage in 1993.

Minutes after 9:03, the principal was back at my open classroom door, her face drawn, clearly pained, and drained of any color. As I walked to her, she met me halfway and took my hand in hers, struggling to keep her feelings under control.

She whispered, "Another plane just crashed into the other tower."

Clasping her hand tighter, I gasped, "We're under attack."

She cleared her throat and said, "I know. Just get the children together, and wait for my instructions."

We hugged and separated, each needing to focus as best we could on the children.

My initial response to the news of the first tower being hit was one of disbelief. After the next plane crashed into the second tower, I knew my city, New York, was under attack. I could only imagine the horror to come.

Calling Juana to my side, I quietly told her what had happened.

"Another plane crashed into the other tower. We're under attack and should to be ready to leave the building if need be."

Her eyes widened as she clutched her throat with both her hands and said, "Oh no, I can't believe it." Then, she lowered her eyelids and began to pray ever so softly.

My thoughts turned to the safety of my own family. Frantic to know whether Matthew and Jodi were safe, I called their home from my classroom, using my cell phone. Jodi was asleep when she answered the phone.

"Thank God, you're home," I cried. "Where's Matthew? Terrorists have attacked the Twin Towers. I can't reach him."

Stunned, she cried, "Oh no, he said that he was going to be downtown, near the Trade Center this morning."

All I could say was, "Please find Matthew."

Where was my son? Was he hurt? Had debris from the shattered planes hit him? Was he unconscious somewhere, ignored by frightened people who struggled to get away from the disaster?

I wanted to run from school to find him but could not until all the children in my care were safe. For me to be trapped and powerless was hard to accept. My stomach tightened with worry as I started to sweat. Where was my son?

Within twenty-five minutes, Jodi called back to say that Matthew was safe but shaken, and he and thousands of others were staggering home across the Brooklyn Bridge.

"Jodi, call me when you finally see him. I love you." Holding back my tears, I wondered if our city's bridges and tunnels would be targeted next. There was no way to know.

Out in the school corridor, confused and shocked staff members hurried about. We nodded to each other but had few words to exchange. How could we have known that on September 11, 2001, we'd experience the most dreadful, horrendous blow ever to strike our country?

On this day, evil men with twisted minds had marked New York City as the site for mass destruction and would take perverse delight in this slaughter of innocents. In seconds, a still autumn sky became animated with flames, clouded by smoke, choking the air with the sickening smell of lives dissolved.

Juana and I did our best not to panic as we prepared the children for what we soon learned would be an early dismissal. As one small group of children finished their breakfasts and the rest sat on the floor scanning through picture books, we quietly removed all clothing and backpacks from their cubbies and placed them behind each child's seat.

When done, I directed my attention back to my class and continued to lead them in our regular morning routines, thereby extending their stability and peace for but a few more minutes. Soon enough, they would learn of the day's tragedies. Surely, all of them would be frightened by the unfathomable, and for weeks to come, many would have nightmares.

By 10:30, both the South and North Tower had collapsed. We were living a tragedy, something that had happened to others, in faraway places, whose names one could barely pronounce, but never to us.

The Board of Education followed the mayor's directive to dismiss all children early from school and made citywide announcements for parents to immediately retrieve their children.

I prayed that our students' families would not suffer the loss of a loved one. To think how frightened and heartbroken a child would be, waiting for a parent he or she would never see again was crushing.

Fortunately within an hour, dazed or alarmed mothers or fathers claimed their children from my class. They had little to say, but I wished them well and cautioned them to be mindful of how upsetting the day's news could be for their children.

My advice to them, "Keep them close, and reassure them that they are safe. Try to distract them from the news on TV and busy them with stories or games. Do the best you can."

Finally dismissed from our responsibilities, Juana and I had hugged each other, relieved to be able to leave school. Suddenly, my cell phone rang. It was Jodi. With my hand shaking, I flipped it open and held it to my ear.

She sobbed, "Matthew just came home."

Without another word of goodbye to anyone, I rushed out the front door of the school but stopped short at the top of its steps, struck still by the beauty of the day. Here, the air had remained fresh, calm, and clear. Cars were still parked along the street. Houses were unchanged, and dogs barked. To believe that disaster had struck only minutes away was difficult.

Shaking my head in disbelief, I began to make my way through a small crowd of parents and children, who were mulling about in front of the school. Those who knew me called out and wished me well, others stopped me to tell me that they were afraid to go home, confused as to what they should do. Without stopping, I counseled them that in time, all would be sorted out. What else could I say?

Finally, I reached my car, opened the door, and sat down to cry. My stomach ached and my head throbbed as my body shook with fear. Today was surreal; it was a bad dream come to life, one without guarantees of what else was to come. I was angry, scared, and grateful that Matt was safe, but God only knew what he had experienced.

Before starting my car I stopped sobbing and called Maxie to tell her Matt and Jodi were all right.

"Maxie, Matthew and Jodi are safe. I am on my way to his house now. Have you heard from Dad? Did he get home?"

"He and his driver just pulled into the driveway. How they managed to get out of the city, I have no idea. Call me later; go to Matthew and Jodi. Be careful. I love you."

Turning on my car, I began the fifteen-minute drive to Matt and Jodi's house in downtown Brooklyn. Theirs was a large, red brick carriage house, complete with stable doors and a domed skylight, located on a beautiful, tree-lined street, anchored with stately brownstones. It stood across the East River from lower Manhattan and the fallen Twin Towers.

The streets were filled with people of all ages moving quickly in all directions. No one laughed, and many were in tears. Cars darted about trying to get from here to there in record time, but no car horns were blown.

Moving closer to Jodi and Matthew's home, the clear air began to change into an eerie, whitewashed gray, filled with tiny particles of dust. It reminded me of fog, rolling noiselessly in to limit visibility.

I parked across the street from their driveway, and saw that Matthew and Jodi were seated on the ground in front of their house folded into each other. Covered in ash, he was slumped against his front door. She was cuddled next to him with her head in his lap, sobbing.

Crying with relief that they were safe and visibly well, I rushed out from my car and fell to the ground to hug and kiss them both. The stories would come later, but for now, I gave thanks that we'd been spared.

Huddled together, we watched as people, clearly shocked, walked past us in the street, as we listened to the screams of ambulance sirens rushing to help the fallen. It was all so terrifyingly sad.

Earlier, Jodi's nursing supervisor had called to ask her to return to St. Luke's Roosevelt Hospital, to be ready to help care for victims of the day's attacks. The city would provide vehicles to transport all critical responders to various locations as needed. With Matthew safe at home, she'd agreed to go.

Knowing Jodi would be gone within the hour, I turned to Matthew. "Do you want me to stay with you?" I touched my hand to his forehead, which was still covered with ash.

I'd already heard about the tragedy of people jumping from the burning towers, of the thousands killed in the flaming skyscrapers, and of survivors outrunning the enormous volcanic-looking plume flooding through the streets. One could only guess as to what Matthew had seen and survived.

Matthew coughed persistently until Jodi ran for a glass of water. He drank it down and managed to whisper, "As soon as Jodi is safely on her way to work, I'm going to shower and sleep. It was horrendous, Mom." He looked at me with sorrow I'd never seen in his eyes. "I'll call if I need you. I promise."

Reluctantly kissing them goodbye, I made my way back to my car and began to drive home. The streets had become all but deserted.

The air became clearer the farther away I drove from downtown. By the time I reached my home, it was once again pristine, which made it harder to believe that such a horrific event had occurred this morning.

Unbelievably, nothing here had physically changed. Safe inside my own home, I called Maxie. Hearing my voice, she broke down and cried.

"How are Matthew and Jodi? I am afraid to call. I'm too nervous," she managed.

"All things considered, they are okay," I lied, but it was a lie of kindness. There was no need for me to terrorize her at this moment. Tomorrow would be a better time to be more forthcoming.

"Maxie, it's been a very long day. I need to shower. Call me later?"

"Okay, but why don't you come to me? I have a refrigerator full of food and I bet you have nothing in yours."

For the first time that day I smiled, pleased by the predictability of her agenda. Family and food, what else was there?

"I'll call you later, Maxie, I need to clean up."

After showering, I sat down in the den and turned on the television. My relief at being alive was tempered by the overwhelming loss of so many in a matter of minutes. Like countless others, I watched television, transfixed by its unrelenting coverage of the city's greatest tragedy.

Film of the towers' collapse was repeated over and over again. It broke my heart to watch them fall and then see the hundreds of people fleeing north on West Street, trying to outrun the deadly ball of smoke and dust that formed as the buildings crashed down.

To acknowledge those who had lost their lives, I tried to read the ensuing obituaries daily, needing to know who they were, rather than just the invisible numbers they'd become. So many of them had survived personal tragedy, only to be brought down, the victims of time and place.

My prayers for the souls and families of those who'd perished seemed futile. It was difficult to justify space for my personal trials. Humbled by a world gone mad, I'd become an insignificant speck.

The staggering events of 9/11 exploded into my mix of emotional turmoil and uncertain health. Sobered by this horrific strike against all sensibilities, it was understood that unlike the innocents who'd perished tragically that day, I had a chance to fight my assailant.

In addition, I experienced a connection to those who, like me, were trying to cope with the sudden and shocking unpredictability of their lives. For me, as for many of us, each step forward was painful to take, but the need to move forward was far greater than the pull backward.

My strength and inspiration came from the citizens of my city, who refused to be broken, and permitted me to continue on. In truth, an opportunity had been granted to me to renew my faith in my ability to appreciate the potential richness of my life. It was a chance to redefine my soul and find refuge from a world changed. To not accept that my life had been deeply altered could lock me into a world of frozen memories.

Cancer had attacked my body and challenged me in my entirety to face my life as it was, and to decide whether to self immolate or rise again.

CHAPTER TWENTY-FOUR

September 18, 2001 – June 2004
Lockdown

Without delay, an armed and highly visible National Guard descended upon the city. Strategically placed, these troops stopped to search vehicles of interest before each entered the city's tunnels, bridges, and select streets.

To both limit and monitor vehicle traffic in and out of Manhattan, no person could drive alone. A necessity of the times, it was an inconvenience accepted without too many complaints.

Under threat of additional terror attacks, the police force increased its presence in subway cars and on station platforms. Amid rumors of impending assaults, trains were often stopped mid-route, which forced passengers to scurry from train to train like rats in a maze.

Traumatized by the colossal destruction of September 11, New Yorkers remained unnaturally subdued under a virtual blanket of anguish. Impromptu memorials appeared throughout the city in the days following the attack. Filled with bouquets of ever-changing flowers, many were illuminated by slow-burning candles, which lit the hundreds of touching notes and drawings placed there to express overwhelming grief. Set alongside these tokens of sorrow were pictures of those still missing, put there in the hope that someone would recall seeing them, somewhere, anywhere.

The need to be close to our loved ones prompted many of us to reach out to them more frequently. Parents walked their children, old and young, to school. Unsure of anything, their goodbyes were often long and emotional. In turn, many students were nervous and confused by the drama they had experienced, made all the more difficult by the stress of heightened vigilance.

Badly shaken by the terrorists' attack, Maxie needed to keep her brood close. During my lunch breaks, I would often walk the one long block from my school to her house. Sitting in her den, we watched the all-consuming news that centered on the attack. Both of us struggled to grasp what had happened on September 11, but neither of us could absorb the enormity of the number of lives lost or comprehend the degree of hatred felt for our country.

Slowly, Matt regained his emotional strength, but he remained distant and depressed, angered over the immense loss of life. Summoned to her hospital to treat survivors of the attack, Jodi and countless other medical personnel still reeled from the reality that so many were beyond their help.

Many times after work, I'd bring them some special wine, cheese, or fruit. Afterward, alone, together, or with one or the other, I'd walk to one of the makeshift memorials that had sprung up on the Brooklyn Heights Promenade. Just blocks from their home, it balanced above the Brooklyn Queens Expressway. Yards away from the East River, it provided a clean view of lower Manhattan.

Gathered to mourn, many visitors to the site remained silent. Others spoke in whispers, as if the recent tragedy had snatched away their voices. A miserable few shuffled about, holding the photo of a missing loved one. To anyone who'd listen, they'd ask, "Do you know them? Have you seen them? Please help me find them."

One evening, a middle-aged woman crumpled into my arms after I'd answered no to her question, "Have you seen my son?"

She leaned heavily on me as I led her to a nearby bench. Seated next to me, she laid her head on my shoulder. Together, we watched the still thick, black smoke spiral up from Ground Zero, which days ago had been converted into a massive funeral pyre.

Slight of build, this woman wore a simple, flower-printed shirt. A soft pink shawl clung to her shoulders and covered some of her long, black hair. Pale under the last of a summer tan, her face was drawn. She could have been me, I she.

Speaking barely above a murmur, she said, "I know my son is dead, but I keep looking for him anyway. I'm not ready to accept that he's gone. My husband is home watching the television. He just sits and cries."

Before taking a long and sad, sad breath, she hugged me gently and stood up. Then, she mouthed, "Thank you."

There was nothing I could say as I watched her walk away. She and thousands of others faced a lifetime of mourning. The only rationale for their loss was unrestrained malevolence.

From within the city and across the country, hundreds came forward to help in any capacity needed. At the crash site, volunteers clawed through the wreckage, many using their bare hands.

The initial program was to rescue victims, hoped to be still alive, in the remaining rubble of melted steel. Slowly and with great sorrow, this plan became a respectful attempt to recover bodies or parts for later identification.

Wounded by this epic disaster, I was eager to physically connect with the event, to be at Ground Zero, but still weak from surgery and adjusting to new medications, I could do no more than volunteer at the Red Cross Command Center, located in Brooklyn at the foot of its namesake bridge.

My assignment: Schedule volunteers who wished to assist at Ground Zero. Countless did so without reservation, but unfortunately, without regard to the greater need, others tried to dictate their terms of service. Displeased by their misguided sense of self, I'd often put them on interminable hold, or better still, disconnect them.

Most faded away, but a tenacious few would repeatedly redial, lost in the selfish dialogue of one, as did a member of the human resource department of a large company.

My conversation with him began well, with no hint of what would follow. He offered at least twenty-five volunteers to help, as they were needed. It was a generous offer, but before I could list the time slots when they could work, he began to state the first of his demands.

"I want all of my people to work side by side. I want them to be as close to Ground Zero as is possible." I said nothing; I knew he could only become more obnoxious in his demands. He continued. "They will be wearing shirts with our company's logo. I will send our staff photographer along to capture pictures of them working."

He then paused for a minute and asked, "Are you listening? Are you writing this down? I want an answer now."

I replied, "It will be impossible to meet your needs and wants. You cannot turn September 11 into a photo op and free advertisement for your company."

He stammered, "This is a very important company, and I have to—"

"No," I said. "All you have to do is hang up the phone."

To be closer to Ground Zero, on more than one occasion, I crossed the Brooklyn Bridge to lower Manhattan. As I looked north, the city remained comfortably the same. Bridges and buildings were in place. Cars moved uptown along East River Drive. To the south, the highway was empty, save for emergency vehicles traveling to and from the demolished World Trade Center.

In Manhattan, I stopped at Chambers street. From there, I could see part of what remained of the collapsed towers: wrecked, twisted pieces of steel. Witnessing this force of pure evil never got easier. Life had become unceasingly sad for us all, not only as individuals but also as citizens of a country devastated by death and destruction.

Cancer, surgery, and September 11 had propelled me to a delicate space between life and death. Much like a marionette, I came to life only when someone pulled my strings. Unsteady, I stood on ground ready to crumble.

For weeks, much of what surrounded me had been threatening. Each day, I'd struggled to crawl out from within my self-imposed cell but was less than successful. Medication, fatigue, and depression governed my life. With one tired step after the other I moved through each day, grateful for the distraction of work and the support of my family and friends.

Within this context, five weeks after my surgery, the second phase of my breasts' reconstruction began: saline injections to be administered by Dr. S in his office on a weekly basis.

Tense and vulnerable, I was one of the many who'd come to the doctor with body parts perceived to be less than perfect; caused by either a genetic disorder, disease, accident, or most often a very personal discontent, patients were optimistic that Dr. S. would transform them into their individual best.

This would be only my third visit to the doctor's office. Initially, I'd walked through his door as a stranger with breast cancer, facing major surgery, depressed and frightened. My second visit was post operation. Now, I was set to move forward with breast reconstruction but was still depressed and sad, now also mourning the loss of lives in the September 11 attacks.

Not to be left behind, Maxie came with me for the first go-round of injections. Though her presence was appreciated, it did nothing to ease my sense of vulnerability.

Wordlessly, I took her hand as I wiped tears from my eyes. Just as she moved closer to put her arm around my shoulder, a nurse appeared and silently motioned to me to follow her.

As I stood up to leave, Maxie began to lift herself up to come with me. Gently, I put my hand on her shoulder and said, "I'll be fine."

Inside the examination room, the nurse handed me a soft robe and said, "Please, put this on with the opening to the front." Reading the sad mix of emotions on my face she said, "You'll be fine. You're exhausted, and rightfully so, but you're heading into the homestretch now."

Hoping to be spared more pain I asked, "Will this procedure hurt?"

She answered, "There should be no pain."

Dr. S walked into the room and greeted me with a wide smile. After a brief examination of my breasts, he lifted his eyes and said, "You're just fine. Today should be easy, but as your chest muscles begin to stretch into your breast cavity, you may experience some discomfort. Everybody responds differently. Just lay back and breathe."

I did as was instructed, but within seconds, I opened my eyes to see, hovering above me, two needles, each long enough to skewer my breasts against the table. I gushed, "Oh my, I'm going to die," and quickly shut my lids. I could hear the doctor and his nurse laugh at my reaction.

"Marjorie, I promise that you will not die on my table today."

As the saline was introduced into each tissue expander, I felt pressure at the injection sites, followed with a rush of pain. When the needles were withdrawn, the doctor said, "Go home and rest."

My breasts hurt, and I was eager to get home to bed, but Maxie insisted we needed to eat, more to sustain a degree of normalcy than from any real hunger on her part.

After I'd dressed and scheduled my next appointment, we walked one block to Madison Avenue to find a quick bite. Small and French, the restaurant we chose held the promise of fine, hot onion soup.

Maxie looked terrible, small, and fragile. Her face was drawn as if she'd not slept well for weeks. She brushed a strand of hair from her face and said, "I don't know how you have the strength to get up each day and walk out the door. This is not the life I want for you."

"Maxie, I don't want this to be my life either. It's difficult to get through each day, but I must be grateful to have the day. You can't control my health and happiness. No one can. It's just what it is."

The soup finally arrived at our table, but proved to be cold and all but inedible. The sandwich we'd added to our order was nothing special. Disappointed, Maxie pushed back against her chair and put her head in her hands. After a long minute, she took a deep breath, lifted her face and smiled.

"Enough of this crap, let's go to Atlantic City this weekend. We need to have some fun."

"What time will you pick me up?" was my answer.

CHAPTER TWENTY-FIVE

Cocktails

My pain was most concentrated immediately after each set of saline injections. Sore all the time, I felt as if I were undergoing orthodonture of my chest, but instead of metal wires being tightened to pull crooked teeth into line, saline was injected into my tissue expanders to stretch my chest's muscles further into my breast cavity.

The reality of my cancer had created fear within me. The 9/11 bombings generated feelings of anger and sorrow. Reconstruction and cancer therapy drugs produced pain and exhaustion. All contributed to my inability to sleep.

Determined for a respite, Ambien and vodka became my cocktail of choice. Mixing alcohol and drugs didn't mean that much to me. I already had cancer. This mix of feel-goods did not make me high, or happy, but did allow me to enjoy at least four hours of uninterrupted sleep.

Each night, at about one o' clock in the morning, I'd pour vodka into a tall glass and slowly count one, two, three, four, and five. With the glass more than half full, I topped it off with cranberry juice, ice, and limes.

With drink in hand, I would carefully walk back to my bedroom to put the radiant cocktail next to my bottle of Ambien, which rested on the table beside my bed.

Smiling at how lovely they looked side by side, I'd slip into a comfortable nightgown and crawl into bed. Not wanting to fall asleep too early and wake up with night hours to spare, I slowly sipped my potion. Each swallow was smooth. I lay back on my pillows and enjoyed the warmth that moved through my body.

Within a half hour, I washed down my Ambien with a final sip. Confident that I would be asleep within minutes, I laid my head back down and closed my eyes.

CHAPTER TWENTY-SIX

Trains

Perceptively slowed under the heavy weight of grief, the battered city would not be brought to its knees. Determined to validate ourselves, we New Yorkers embraced our ability to go beyond the heinous acts committed against us on September 11. Throughout this time, it became necessary for me to continue to visit both my oncologist and plastic surgeon. As the single occupancy car laws were in now in effect,my travel to and from Manhattan would be achieved via the subway.

Having successfully avoided the underground system for years, this would be a tremendous challenge to me. Uncomfortable among crowds, I was too nervous to be standing on a station platform amid hundreds of people. My need to see the day's light always made me anxious.

Sensing my distress, Jodi graciously volunteered to go with me on what would be my first train ride in a very long while. It would end with a visit to my oncologist in Manhattan.

With a ceremonious double-swipe of her metro card one rainy morning, Jodi and I set out to ride the rails.

I tried hard to relax, but I could do nothing more than sit close by Jodi's side, safe in her company. With eyes wide, I tried to imprint the stations we passed in my mind so I could get back home. Too nervous to remember anything, after three or four, I gave up. When we reached our destination, Jodi asked, "Do you still have your train token?" Feeling the piece in my pocket, I smiled in answer.

We trudged the block to the oncologist's office. Within minutes, I was seen by my oncological nurse, and the doctor, as well. Blood drawn, pressure taken, glands felt. My visit was over.

Jodi and I put on our jackets and left the office. Once we were outside, prepared to go our separate ways, she again asked, "Do you still have the token?"

Nodding yes, I proudly pulled it from my pocket to show her. I laid it across my open palm, and said, " Look, it's not lost."

As I ended my prideful declaration, Jodi and I watched in horror as the token rolled from my hand and fell directly into the subway grate below. In shock, we looked at each other and laughed.

"Typical me," I said.

Jodi had to attend a meeting across town, but first she walked me to the subway entrance. Reassuring her that I could manage on my own, we kissed goodbye. As I watched her rush to the bus stop, my eyes filled with tears.

Forced now to buy my own metro card, I proceeded to swish it and myself into the Holy Land of Rolling Rumbles.

Encouraged by having survived that first train ride, I continued to take the subway to and from Manhattan.

With a small waist pack hidden beneath my clothes, much of the time I felt like Stanley in search of Livingston, Hillary scaling Mt. Everest, or Lawrence crossing Arabia as I trekked north, south, east, and west, uptown, downtown, cross town, and back.

For me to get anywhere underground was a real challenge. I had to concentrate so I wouldn't be swept along by the many people racing about, who seemed unassailable thanks to their anonymity.

I often wondered who among them possessed a dark and terrible secret. Had any of my fellow travelers lost a loved one on 9/11? Was the man standing at the train's door trapped by personal tragedy, or was he one of "them" and going to blow up the train? Did the middle-aged woman standing next to me have breast cancer?

I'd taken my last train ride at least thirty years before. In that time, the subway had changed a great deal. Many of the city's teenagers ran amok, unsupervised, without self-control. Conversations between passengers were often annoyingly loud. Crowded just shy of overfilling, seats were prized and not given up if ever attained.

The subway had become a veritable underground bazaar; people now carried everything and anything onto the trains. Food, strollers, furniture, anonymous packages of every description, and all seemingly in multiples of ten, were in sight.

Some fellow riders were industrious. Among my favorites were those who'd attached all sorts of sundry items to their bodies. By doing this, they'd transformed themselves into self-contained mini variety stores. Many wore amusing hats with propellers attached to their tops. Perhaps they were secret decoders that allowed them to coordinate their portfolios.

Terrorists had assaulted our sensibilities and made us nervous. At any hint of "police activity," the trains were delayed. No one really knew what "activity" meant, and this unknown primed the collective imaginations of subway riders to run wild.

Easily disoriented by the subway's inherently complicated system, more often than not, I became lost. Seeing the panic in my eyes and hearing the anxiety in my voice, most of the travelers were kind and helpful, which only reinforced the fact that New Yorkers are the most generous of souls in times of need. I always returned home safe and sound, although many times I arrived there much later than I'd planned.

Looking back on my underground adventures, I can proudly say I was sung to, shoved against, cursed at, and best of all, flirted with on more than one occasion.

At last, I had become a real New Yorker.

CHAPTER TWENTY-SEVEN

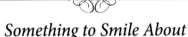

Something to Smile About

After the third go round of injections, I noticed that my bosom had become significantly larger, the curves of my body more clearly defined. Less red, raised, and angry, my surgical scars were finally retreating into fine horizontal lines. My missing nipples created a strange esthetic, not unpleasant to me.

For me to find a comfortable spot on which to rest my expanding breasts was quite the challenge. Lying on my stomach made me feel as if I were suspended on two water balloons. Resting on my side left me at a loss as to where to place my arms. Should they go above my head, under my chin, or close to my side? Had I been cursed with two pairs of arms and four breasts?

Relishing these changes as a sign of moving forward, I began to re-evaluate the ultimate goal of my reconstruction. Surgery had permanently altered my body; to embrace this change would be positive. Perhaps becoming a 36C, rather than a whisper of a 34B, could be the lift I needed.

After each treatment, I'd leave Dr. S's office and then turn the corner to walk downtown along Park Avenue until I reached East 86th street. From there, I'd make my way to Lexington Avenue and take the subway home.

Throughout that October, the weather had remained mild. Wearing a light sweater was more than enough, and leaving it unbuttoned made it easier for me to steal quick, sideways peeks at my bosom in any mirrors or closed windows I passed.

On one particularly exquisite late afternoon, after I'd said my goodbyes to the doctor and his staff, I stopped short in front of a large, glass-sided wall and caused a stroller, pushed too close behind me, to be run up my leg.

Unharmed, I mumbled, "Sorry," to the nanny but stood my ground, riveted by my reflection. After she'd nodded and rolled around me, I turned and faced my mirrored image full on. For the first time in a very long while, I saw my own smile. I blinked my eyes several times and shook my head to see if it was a fluke.

The smile fixed on my face again signaled to me that I'd come far enough along in my recuperation and reconstruction to begin to focus on my future. Within weeks, I would choose which implants would replace my tissue expanders.

Although Marlo and I had qualified and quantified a good number of breasts in Italy, I wanted to know the results of Mutt's research. Even though we'd spoken daily, I'd not seen him since his visit almost six weeks ago. I called him that evening and learned that he'd been working on a business model.

He suggested we meet the upcoming Saturday afternoon. "You and I will have some fun with this," he said. "I've been waiting for you to ask me and hoped it wouldn't be as long as I've waited to sleep with you."

I laughed, answering, "I'll give you half your wish."

As I dressed to meet Mutt, I chose my clothes thoughtfully, knowing that he would observe every detail. A close-to-the bone, simple T-shirt minimized the still uneven plane of my breasts. A totally clear palette would be unattainable without wearing a bra, which I could not do until my reconstruction was complete.

I pulled on a pair of slim, black jeans, and covered my feet with black ballet flats. Secured by only two buttons, a soft pink cardigan. New, it was a delicious cover and a reward for my trials. I pulled my hair back into a ponytail and kept my makeup simple.

We met at the same bistro where we'd initially discussed my project. Again, seated with his back against the brick wall, he had a full view of the entire café, as well as the street beyond.

In response to the cooler weather, instead of wrapping his silver-gray V-necked sweater around his shoulders, he'd pulled it over a black T-shirt, which matched his pressed dungarees. Dark sunglasses covered his eyes.

To watch the smile on his face broaden whenever I approached him was always a treat. But today, the foot traffic outside distracted him, and I was denied his warm look of expectation.

As I neared the table, I could see a slew of photos and magazines next to his half-open briefcase. It was obvious that he had done his homework well.

Still unnoticed, I leaned in very close to his body, placed one hand lightly on his back, and brushed my lips across his cheek. Then I whispered, "May I join you?"

Taken completely off guard, he fell back against the bricks. As he jumped up to face me, his sunglasses fell to the floor. He also managed to smash his leg against the table with such force that all the photos and his briefcase crashed to the floor.

Unaccustomed to seeing him lack control of anything, I laughed hard and long and stopped only to give him a quick hug. We both got down on our hands and knees to collect his scattered materials. As we scooped up the bits, I noticed that every piece of material reflected the image of a fabulous-looking woman with exquisite breasts, some covered, some not.

We sat down after we'd picked everything up. I was more than ready to listen to his presentation, but instead he declared, "We need our strength; let's get something to eat."

"Okay, let's share the mussels in garlic and wine, and I'll have a glass of Pinot Grigio."

After the waiter had taken our order, Mutt looked at me and said, "You look great, but tell me little one, how do you really feel?"

"Well, my friend, I feel better than I have in a long while, although I'm still reeling from September 11. My medicines beat me up every day. I have almost no energy, but I'm excited about my implants." Taking a breath I added, "Most important, I'm smiling again."

He returned my smile, and said, "You know, I've missed that smile."

"Me too."

After the waiter had brought our food, I watched as Mutt soaked up the wine sauce with pieces of thick, crusted bread. As he relished each bite, I drank my wine and recalled my initial visit to Dr. S's office.

After we'd finished eating, Mutt twisted his graceful hand and motioned for the waiter to clear and clean the table. Mutt reopened his briefcase on the now-spotless surface and spread before me images of absolutely gorgeous women.

Nodding to me, he answered, "I think implants filled with silicone, rather than saline, are more appealing, visually, and feel more natural to the touch."

Size, to him, was of little consequence. He bowed to the aesthetics created by a well-defined bosom, proportionate to the body, as long as there was a balance and symmetry of line.

To illustrate this point, he took out a pencil and a piece of paper from his briefcase and began to illustrate how a woman with too large a bosom would fall over face first, weighed down beyond her control. With a flourish, he wrote "Splat" underneath the picture.

My smile encouraged him to continue to draw. The second figure sported very small—tiny—breasts. With the pencil's eraser, he next rubbed the figure into obscurity.

Pleased with his demonstration, he winked at me and said, "Too little is just a waste."

We decided that my future implants would be larger than oranges, smaller than cantaloupes and definitely filled with silicone. Our conference at an end, we toasted my forthcoming bosom with a clink of his water glass against the rim of my wine goblet.

CHAPTER TWENTY-EIGHT

Implants

Being excited about yet another surgical procedure seemed odd, but the thought of having my tissue expanders removed and replaced with silicone breast implants the coming morning had me in high spirits. After that, all that remained of my breasts' reconstruction would be the rebuilding of my nipples.

Maxie had wanted to come with me, but when I told her that tomorrow's weather was dialed into lousy and that she would need to get up at 5:00 a.m. she changed her mind. Before swallowing my usual mixture of vodka and Ambien, I called her to say goodnight.

"Goodnight, Maxie, I'll call you when I get back."

"Just take care, I love you."

As the receiver reached its cradle, the phone rang again. Matthew had called to remind me to be ready at 5:00 am.

"Matthew, I sure hope this is the last time you need to take me to the hospital for a long, long time."

"Me too, Mom."

As soon as I'd turned off the phone and stretched out on my bed, a massive cough burst through my ribs and threatened to snatch my heart from my chest. What had begun as a peep three days before had became a roar. With surgery scheduled in the morning, I'd slugged cough medicine all day to rid myself of this beast, or at least contain it. Frantic for relief, I added the medicine to my vodka and washed down my daily dose of Ambien with a final and now fowl sip. Within minutes, I fell asleep.

Without dreams to hold onto, I opened my eyes well before 5:00 a.m. excited to be on my way. I sat up, but almost immediately, my obstinate cough smacked me back down. Panicked at the thought that my surgery would need to be postponed, I ran into the bathroom and turned on the hot water to create some steam. Perhaps it would relieve my distress.

Surrounded by the moist white cloud, I breathed in deeply to relax my muscles. Shortly thereafter, my cough retreated just enough for me to dress quickly and be on time to meet Matthew.

It was a cold, rotten November day and a definitive end to the much-needed nice weather we'd been blessed with directly following the September 11 attacks. Angry pellets of rain attacked me until I slipped into the car, wet all over.

We were not alone on the highway, but as it was still early in the morning, we'd avoided the daily push of traffic into Manhattan. As we neared the Brooklyn Bridge, I could see police positioned at its entrance. Their sober presence had become a permanent response to the September 11 strikes.

As we neared the bridge's approach ramp, my cough staged a reprisal, which forced me to twist and turn to catch my breath. As I squirmed and wheezed, the policeman closest to me leaned toward our car, curious as to my movements. Was I spastic? Was I signaling for help? Was I a threat? If my movements were not controlled, he would surely pull us over to begin a lengthy security check, and I would be dangerously late for my procedure.

At the moment when the officer began to lift his hand to stop us, my cough miraculously retreated long enough for me to manage a wave.

He let us pass.

Midway on the bridge, Matthew turned to me and asked, "Wouldn't it be best for you to cancel the surgery? You're really having a tough time."

Between coughs I answered, "No, I'm just fine."

Of course, Matthew was right; it made me think of how childlike we parents can become, almost to the point of being ridiculous. I was foolhardy and stubborn, but my will to move ahead with my reconstruction overcame logical thoughts.

In good time we reached the hospital. After parking the car, we walked into the hospital and took the elevator to the surgical suite. It would, I hope, be an easy in, easy out, with no bags to carry—nothing but the clothes on my back.

Though no one said it was nice to see me again, the operating room staff greeted me like an old friend. Feeling my cough bubble up again and frightened that I would break into another round of coughing, I feigned nerves and asked for a sedative, thinking that a shot in my bottom was better than being tossed out of surgery. Willingly, the anesthesiologist administered the relaxant, and my cough eased. Before I fell asleep, Matthew's anxious smile registered in my brain. I hoped to see it again soon.

Three hours later, I opened my eyes and saw a nurse leaning over me. Within minutes, Dr. S appeared with a wide smile on his face. "Marjorie, your surgery was a success. Go home, get some rest, and enjoy your beautiful new bosom. See you in my office in two weeks to complete your reconstruction."

With a nurse to help me, I walked back to the locker room. Eager to see and feel what the doctor had crafted, I looked in the mirror before I dressed.

Though covered with small bandages, I could see that each of my breasts had been cut halfway, from outside to midway front. Tentatively touching them, I found them to be firm but soft. Mutt had been on the mark; silicone was terrific. My breasts were lovely.

For just a moment, I bowed my head to give thanks for the success of today's surgery and tried not to dwell on the steps I'd taken to reach this point for fear that I'd fall into a heap of exhaustion.

With sweatshirt in hand, I walked out of the locker area into the room where Matthew had been waiting. He smiled his wonderful smile and leaned close to kiss me. Then, he shot a glance at my breasts, which were covered only with a long-sleeved t-shirt. He nodded his head in approval and said, "Nice." It was all I needed to hear.

He took my arm, and together we walked to the garage across the street.

While we waited for the car, I remembered waking up in the recovery room after my mastectomies. Then, I had felt my son's kiss upon my cheek. Unable to speak to him, I cried. Today, I turned to my loving child and kissed him on his cheek. I did not cry.

We exited the hospital garage and crept into the lunchtime traffic. With my implants intact and my cough still tamed from anesthesia, both Matthew and I were relieved to have the morning's events behind us. Without the pressure to be on time for my appointment, neither of us complained about the crush of cars, slowed more by the unceasing rain.

Still drowsy, I closed my eyes. One hour later, Matthew woke me; we'd reached my home.

I took his hand in mine and said, "Matt, I can go upstairs by myself. It's time for you to leave and get some rest. It's time for you to focus on yourself and Jodi."

"Mom, are you sure?"

"Yes, it's been too much about me these last few months."

I kissed him goodbye and tried without luck to keep dry as I rushed back into my building. Thoroughly soaked, I dripped water onto the lobby floor. Inside my own home, I striped off my clothes and dried off.

Standing in front of my full-length mirror, I looked at my refitted bosom, and then slowly revisited my body's scars, many of which represented an effort to preserve my life.

Each scar reminded me that the human body is transitory, and it must be cherished. Without these scars, I might not have survived to be loved and to love in return. They heralded the resilience of not just my body, but of my soul. I believed that the essence of my beauty was in the life within me, which I was still blessed to share.

Smiling to myself, I turned away and wrapped myself in a warm nightgown. I wanted to call Mutt to share my excitement about my implants, but that could wait until tomorrow. Maxie would not.

She must have been waiting near the telephone, for she answered my call at its first ring.

"Well?" she asked.

"They're magnificent," I told her.

"Get some rest."

"Yes."

Shutting off the phone, I bundled myself into my warm covers, and without my usual cocktail, slept until one the next morning, when impatient to see how my clothes would fit my new silhouette, I got out of bed and pulled everything and anything from my drawers and closets. I let the top of my nightgown drop down around my hips and began to dress and undress, trying on as many pieces of clothing as I could.

Though more than pleased with my appearance, one important test remained: to see if a simple blouse would still fall sadly away from my shoulders and slide down my back. In the past, without a full enough bosom to anchor the shirt in place, it had done so, much to my annoyance.

Selecting a blue oxford shirt, I put it on and slowly closed each button. As I did, I felt an unfamiliar yet reassuring tug of fabric across my breasts. Encouraged, I tucked the shirt's ends into my gown and began to move about the room. It remained in place, which was a small, unexpected gift.

Later in the day, the soreness of my breasts woke me. I touched them tenderly, grateful that they were soft, supple, and cancer free. Compared with the pain after my mastectomies, my discomfort was minimal and could be managed without prescription drugs.

I pushed up from the bed, lowered my feet to the floor and felt them rub against something silky. Looking down, I saw they'd touched a favorite blouse, now twisted and turned. Close by, skirts and pants were piled into a heap as other pieces of clothing dangled dangerously from their hangers.

My bedroom was a mess, created when I'd tried on most of my clothes. Before weeding through this jumble, I checked my phone messages. There were five. Marlo and Ava were calls one and two. Mutt owned calls three, four, and five. Clearly annoyed that he hadn't heard from me, his messages were colorful. His would be returned first.

Not waiting for him to finish saying "Hello," I jumped in and said, "Mutt, I love my implants."

With the swiftness of a machine gun, he shot back, "Glad it worked out for you, but you should have called me sooner. What is the matter with you? Do you think I don't care? I have a lot invested in you, Baby Girl."

When he took a breath to arm himself with more words, I replied, "Did you ever think that I was tired after my procedure and might need to sleep?"

Instead of launching a counter attack, he sighed. "Let's move on. I was worried. I hate hospitals. When do I get to see your breasts? I deserve a private showing."

Relieved that he'd calmed down, I joined in the fun. "I suppose you want a special lap dance from me as well?"

Laughing hard, he said, "That would be nice, but it's not quite all that I've wished from you."

"Since you're less than satisfied with my offer, it's now off the table."

"I'm wounded. At least give me some hope that we will couple before we die."

"It will happen."

He interrupted me mid-thought and said, "Okay, how about having brunch this Sunday at Azul on Stanton Street at one o'clock? I love you."

"Love you more. I will be there. Goodbye."

Mutt would speak his mind without prompts, which would make his unfiltered reaction to my implants interesting. Though too passionate about most everything, he'd lately been higher strung than usual, which undoubtedly wreaked havoc on his worn and fragile heart.

I'd never given up urging him to "Be careful, relax, and take a break." Silence was his consistent response.

After my conversation with Mutt, and before I had time to go to the bathroom, Maxie called. "Marjorie, I'm coming to see you right now. I must see your implants."

"Sure Max, come as soon as you can."

Within fifteen minutes, Maxie rang my doorbell. Weighed down by a large bag filled with groceries, she walked straight into my kitchen. Usually her driver did the heavy lifting, but today she wanted me all to herself.

As soon as she put her bag down on the counter, she turned to me and said, "Well?"

I smiled, unbuttoned my shirt, and bared my breasts. She inhaled deeply, closed her eyes for a minute, then opened them and looked straight at my bosom. I placed her hands lightly on my breasts so that she could feel how soft they were.

With tears rolling down her cheeks, she raised her hands and cradled my face, then stepped back and said, "They're beautiful."

As I buttoned my shirt, she dried her tears with the backs of her hands and said, "I was so furious that I couldn't make your cancer go away, I all but denied that you had it at all. In my heart, it was obvious that you'd made the right decision to undergo mastectomies, but not being able to do more for you frustrated me so damn much."

"Maxie, you've done enough."

She washed her face at the sink, then turned to me and smiled with a twinkle in her eye. Then, as if planned, we both said, "Let's eat."

In two days, my room was in order, I felt well, and looked forward to dinner with Ava and Marlo that evening.

During my weeks at home, they'd made it a point to cheerfully chauffeur me to dinner or the movies, even though my fatigue could short-circuit the evening.

Marlo and Ava arrived together, quickly followed by the food I'd ordered. It was steaming hot, so we worked quickly to empty each container into serving dishes and set them on my dining room table. Within minutes we sat down to a delicious meal of pasta, veal, eggplant, and chicken. Bottles of wine, red and white, stood ready to be uncorked.

Before a bite or sip was taken, Marlo asked us to join hands and lower our heads. Softly, she said, "God, bless our meal and our friendship. Thank you for delivering Marjorie from cancer. Please keep her safe."

Holding my friends' hands more tightly, I thanked Marlo and Ava for their support. After we dropped our hands, I moved my chair back, stood up, lifted my T-shirt and bared my breasts yet again.

"Ladies, here they are. What do you think?"

"Do they move?" Marlo asked, taking another sip of her wine.

I answered, "Yes," and demonstrated their range of motion with care.

"Can you sleep on them comfortably?" was Ava's next question as she, too, raised her glass, filled with white wine.

"Not yet."

"Can you wear a bra?" Marlo asked.

"Not yet."

"Do you need a bra?" queried Ava.

"No, my breasts are permanently perky."

"When do you get tattooed?" Marlo asked as she refilled her glass with more red wine.

"In three weeks."

"Do they hurt at all?" was Ava's final question, before she finished her first glass of wine.

"Only a very little bit."

Laughing, I covered my bosom and said, "Ladies, let's eat before we have to reheat all this food."

Before they left, I handed them each a ribbon-tied bag filled with some of my clothes, which they'd admired, that no longer fit me.

"Ladies, make your own memories in them."

CHAPTER TWENTY-NINE

Restart

No longer invincible, and vulnerable to being attacked, New Yorkers had become emotional refugees within their city after the horror of September 11, 2001. To see or hear a plane fly overhead made some of us wince, suck in our breath with dread in the expectation that it might explode, crash into a building, or hurl itself to the ground.

Subways, tunnels, and bridges remained guarded by police. Access into public buildings was subject to intense inspections. Cars were stopped, bags checked, and lines at airports grew longer as security checks were conducted.

The painful cleanup at Ground Zero continued as workers judiciously tried to find something, anything, amidst the debris to identify those who'd been burned or crushed to death when the Twin Towers fell.

In the year after the terrorist attacks, my city crawled forward and displayed important signs of healing. Traffic was back to its feverish pace, people shouted and cursed at each other, and restaurants were again full.

To mark the first anniversary of the violence we'd experienced, a memorial service was held at the site of the strike. Hundreds of people gathered there to honor those who'd died during the onslaught, carrying pictures of those they'd lost.

Throughout the moment of silence, the respectful speeches, and the poignant, reverential reading of the names of those who'd perished, was the tacit understanding that a raw, uncontrolled hatred had killed their loved ones and destroyed their lives forever.

Throughout the year, my trials persisted and remained unchanged. Medications still ruled my level of activities. My job left me with little energy for anything else during the workweek. Only on the weekend did I connect with my family and friends.

My visits to the oncologist every three months that first year after surgery were tough. Only after I'd cleared his examination and received news that the blood he'd drawn was negative could I calm my nerves until the next doctor's visit and battery of tests three months later.

Matthew remained distant and withdrawn. Though only the most callous of people could remain unchanged by the attack, I sensed that something beyond shock and anger gnawed at him.

My generic questions were inadequate. The hugs and kisses I used to soothe him as a little boy were now inappropriate. Not wanting to intrude on his grief made it hard for me to comfort him.

In Jodi, Matt had a loving partner, which gave me hope that in time he would be able to put planks over these emotional holes and lift himself up.

One Sunday morning, late in October of 2002, as I was getting ready to meet Mutt for brunch, Matt and Jodi called to see if we all could have dinner later in the week. Always eager to spend time with them, I answered quickly. "Of course. Let me know where and at what time."

Time!

I looked at my clock and realized I was going to be late for my brunch with Mutt. He would be counting the minutes on his watch, but I would blame it on traffic and smile. It usually worked.

Hot-tempered and quick-witted, my friend demanded that his life be anything but colorless. I'd loved him forever but, intimidated by his strength of purpose, I'd contented myself to be his beloved friend, comforted by his presence.

Throughout my health upheaval, he'd become even more attentive and needed daily reassurance that I was doing well. Perhaps my illness jarred the memory of his own dramatic surgery, or perhaps something else motivated him to be more demonstrative toward me, but either way, it remained a puzzle. For now, all I could manage to do was to let our relationship continue as an uncomplicated comfort. With that thought in mind, I went to my car and drove into Manhattan to meet him.

Fortunately the single occupancy restriction on cars driving into Manhattan had been lifted, and within fifteen minutes, I parked my car a short block from the restaurant. I turned the corner and saw that Mutt stood outside the bistro. After he saw me, he rushed to me, grabbed my hand, and spun me around.

"Well, hello to you, too," I said.

"Okay, okay, kiss, kiss, and all that, I made reservations for us around the corner, and we're late," he said as he propelled me along the busy street. Strange, Mutt rarely made reservations.

We stopped in front of a small storefront that displayed at least ten different varieties of salami next to a basket full of pate, bread, and cheese. Bottles of oil, vinegar, and wine lined the remainder of the window.

Mutt moved me inside and said, "Ciao, ci scusi, il trafico."

A short, round man walked from behind the counter, smiled at us, and said, "Non c'e` problema." He shook Mutt's hand and guided us through his cluttered shop to its backyard.

The small outdoor space had been transformed into a lush garden. A large oak tree anchored the area, along with small fruit trees bearing figs and lemons. Flowers in shades of purple, pink, red, orange, and yellow melded together in a rainbow of color.

Beneath the oak tree was a small table covered with a red checked cloth. Two wicker chairs flanked either side. It was set for two with colorful dishes, napkins, and utensils. Standing guard, two goblets waited to be filled with wine.

Amazed at the unexpected, I started to laugh with excitement as Mutt pulled out a chair and nodded for me to sit down. Before I could ask the question, he answered, "We have a lot to celebrate."

With a smile on his face, he motioned the owner to begin to serve us brunch. He poured the white wine for me, and then filled one for Mutt, who said defensively, "If I die today, I will die a happy man."

I sat back in my chair, breathed in the sharp autumn air, and let the wine travel down my throat. Even though a small fireplace warmed us, the air remained chilly, and I was glad I'd worn a warm sweater set and winter-weight jeans.

After putting down my glass, I reached over and took Mutt's hand. "Thank you." Warmed by the heat of the fire, I unbuttoned my cardigan.

Mutt looked at my silhouette, threw back his head, then laughed and said, "Baby Girl, they're gorgeous. I cannot believe they're not real. Can I finally feel them now? Six months ago all I got was a quick look."

Feigning shock, I answered, "Is this why you went to the fuss of us having a private meal?"

"Of course. This is an event to be shared only between us," he answered slyly.

Without much internal debate, I answered by standing up and walking directly to him. Taking his hands, I let them feel my breasts.

For just a moment, I saw a flash of surprise before his expression turned to one of pleasure.

Slowly, very, very, slowly, he passed his hands over, around, and between my breasts. I held my breath and, and...one potato, twopotato, how long would this take?

His strong, tapered fingers had stopped to party with my bosom.

Pulling my hand slowly back, I smacked him hard up the side of his head.

Before I pulled away from him, he drew me close and kissed my cheek, not once but twice.

Then he whispered, "I love you and need you to be well."

My answer was to kiss him back, sit down, and take another sip of wine.

We joked and laughed our way through what became an early dinner. The food was as good as anything I'd eaten in Italy. Before desert was served, Mutt pulled a small wrapped box from his jacket and handed it to me without a word. Not knowing what this could mean, I looked at him for a clue and received nothing but a soft command to open it.

Inside was a watch. Stunned, I picked it up and looked closely at its rectangular face. Strong black plus signs replaced the 12, 3, 6, and 9 on its dial.

Mutt whispered, "From today forward, each minute is a plus."

Stunned, I watched as he reached over and fastened the watch to my wrist. "Don't thank me, and please don't cry. We're blessed to be here."

He must have intuited my next question would be, "Why this gift now?" and continued with, "I waited to give this to you because I didn't want to push you." Before I could ask him, "Push me into what?" he waved his hand and signaled for our check.

Within minutes, we'd walked away from our secret garden to sit side by side in my car. Only then did I turn to him and say, "Thank you."

He drew me close and kissed me. Deep and sweet, his kiss was perfect, but within seconds it was over. Still tasting his lips, I caught my breath and smiled.

Mutt started to get out of my car to make his way uptown, but not used to drinking, he was less than steady and sunk back into his seat. Looking straight ahead he said, "Home." And then he closed his eyes.

I pulled his seat belt across his chest, locked the car doors, and drove until I'd double-parked in front of his modern, high-rise building. No longer soothed by the sound of the car's engine, Mutt opened his eyes and muttered in mock annoyance, "No, silly girl, I meant home to your bed."

"You're in no shape to do anything but sleep in your bed, alone."

"Baby Girl, it's been a wonderful day with more to come."

With difficulty, he pulled himself up from his seat and motioned for his building's doorman to open the car door. Just before he left, he touched my arm and said, "I love you."

To his back, I whispered, "I love you, too," and looked down at my watch. I pressed it to my lips and murmured what he had said when he gave it to me. "Plus," he'd said. "From today forward, each day is a plus."

CHAPTER THIRTY

Dinner at Seven

As I watched him walk through the doorway of his building, my cell phone rang. It was Matthew.

"Mom, would you like to meet Jodi and me for a dinner tonight, around seven o'clock, instead of later in the week?"

Though still full from my brunch with Mutt, I said yes immediately. Dinner with Matthew and Jodi was always fun, and as our three schedules rarely gelled, it was all but impossible to make it happen often. This would be a treat.

"Where should we meet?"

"Let's start off with drinks at our house."

It was close to five o'clock, but without a traffic delay on East River Drive, there would be enough time for me to go home, wash my face, rest, and change into a warmer sweater.

The gods smiled; the highway was empty, and I breezed home in twenty minutes. After I'd washed my face and put on a thick, cozy sweater, I lay down on the couch in my den, closed my eyes and mentally replayed my day with Mutt.

My relationship with him was becoming more and more convoluted, but trying to dissect it would serve no purpose. Just getting through each day was difficult enough for me. At the moment, my life did not need another challenge.

At 6:45, I got up from bed, combed my hair, grabbed a jacket, locked my front door and drove to Matt and Jodi's house. After I'd rung their doorbell, Jodi opened the door and leaned down quickly to kiss me without a word. Matt was standing behind her and pulled me into his chest for a gentle hug.

I followed them into their living room and sat down in one of their deep brown leather armchairs. Matthew poured Jodi and me a glass of red wine. On their wood coffee table rested Matthew's half empty glass of scotch.

Jodi seemed unusually quiet; she sat back on the couch with her hands held close together. Her face was strained, and her soft, blue eyes were rimmed in red. Either her allergies had kicked in, or she'd been crying.

Before I could say, "Are you all right?" Matthew served us our drinks and sat down next to her. He put one arm around her shoulder, lifted his glass with the other, and drank the remainder of his of scotch.

He put down his empty glass and faced me without a smile. "Mom, there is no easy way to tell you this."

This? This? What the hell was this? Was one of them sick? Were they going to move? Were they getting a divorce? My gut felt as it had when I was told that I had breast cancer.

Matthew continued. "Mom, after the September 11 attacks, I enlisted as an information officer in the United States Coast Guard Reserves. I'm to report for training next week at Cape May New Jersey and then will be assigned to the Coast Guard facility at Battery Park, in lower Manhattan."

He paused for a minute to collect himself and then said, "In time, I may be heading out to the Persian Gulf for six months." Looking at Jodi, he pulled her close to his side. "It's important to me that I do this. Jodi has mixed feelings, but she's agreed to support me." He ended with, "Mom, I hope you will, too."

Oh my. This was scary—crazy.

Did Matt just tell me that he'd enlisted in the Coast Guard and that he might be going to the Persian Gulf? First cancer smacks me, then my city is attacked on September 11, and now my son may be transported to a foreign country to face any threat deemed dangerous by someone all but anonymous.

It was hard for me not to faint or crumble into a gob of selfish hysteria. I held tightly to the sides of my chair to stop me from falling to my knees to beg Matt to reconsider. Then I thought, a note, I could write a note: "To whom it may concern, you cannot have my son. He cannot go. I, his mother, will not let him go anywhere."

Matt and Jodi watched my every move but said nothing as they waited for me to respond. A fit would serve no purpose. It would surely come later when I was alone, but now I could not lose control. They needed me to be calm. They needed me to be strong, supportive, and stable. I needed to earn an academy award for acting.

"Mom, say something."

"Matt," I whispered, "please get me a real drink."

"Those bastards bombed our city, killed our neighbors. I can't just sit here at home and do nothing," Matt said and handed me a full glass of scotch, as Jodi came to sit on the arm of my chair.

I downed a generous mouthful and followed it quickly with another swig to finish it off. The blast of liquid burned the back of my throat, but the resulted buzz was needed.

My head still hurt, but the alcohol relaxed my body. I managed to take Jodi's hand and say, "May God protect you both."

Matt looked at me, incredulous that I did not jump up, grab his arm and scream, "No, no, no, I refuse to let you go."

He refilled his glass once again, drank a bit and continued softly. "Mom, do you understand what I've just told you?"

Looking at his tired face, I took a breath and answered gently, "Matt, I heard every word you said, but I've also heard every word that Jodi did not speak. It's taking all my strength, and some of your good scotch to not break down.

"You've made your decision. All that's left for me to do is support you both. No parent wants her child to be in harm's way, but we're all just part of something greater than us."

Matt took another sip from his glass and walked to me. With tears in my eyes, I stood up and welcomed him into my arms.

Emotionally drained, we never made it to a restaurant but settled for Thai food delivered to the house.

Initially we ate in silence; our thoughts of the potential ramifications of Matt's enlistment sealed us off from each other. Only after I'd voiced my complaint, "Maxie will blame me for letting Matt join the Armed Forces," did we begin to relax.

"She'll be furious with me when she learns that you've enlisted. It's going to get ugly very quickly."

Matt and Jodi turned to each other and smiled. Maxie's temper was legendary. Never mind that Matt was an adult and married to a strong, intelligent woman. As Matt's mother, I was responsible for him at all times.

Jodi grinned and said, "I'll keep my first aid kit ready. Maxie might chew you up."

Matt added, "If she could cut you up and squeeze you into a blender one limb at a time and spin the blade at low speed, that might make her feel better."

"Thank you both."

"She will be terrified," I added.

" I know," Matt whispered.

I kissed Matt and Jodi, then drove straight home.

At eleven that night the incessant ring of the phone greeted me at the door. Shaky and teary-eyed, I weighed my options—answer it? Or crawl back into the sickbed I'd fought so hard to get out of? There was no doubt who was on the other end of the line. It had to be Maxie.

With every right to be scared, angry, and frustrated she would be at her wits end and want to change Matt's decision to enlist. Without a doubt, our conversation would be difficult, although we surely mirrored each other's fears.

Before I answered the strident, demanding phone, I pulled off my sweater and sat down on the couch in my den. I lifted the receiver, and heard Maxie scream, "Where the hell have you been? You didn't tell me that Matt enlisted in the Coast Guard. He could be going to the Persian Gulf. Why did you let him do this? What the hell is wrong with you? What's wrong with him?"

Without stopping, she added, "His father's dead, and I've almost lost you, but I will not lose him. There is no way in hell that Matt is going to do this."

When she finally paused for a moment, I said softly, "Maxie, I didn't know about this until tonight. I'm as upset as you, but he's made his decision and all we can do is support him."

"Look," she railed, "Matt could..." then she began to sob. "If something happens to him...I just can't think of it."

"Maxie, we're powerless to change his mind."

"I know, but my God, he and Jodi just got married. Can't you do something? You're his mother; how can you be so damned passive about this?"

It took everything inside not to scream back at her, not to slam down the phone, not to call Matt and beg him not to go. It took everything to answer, "I'm frightened, too, but we can't do anything but pray that he will be safe."

There was a long silence, and I put my head in my hand, bracing for another barrage from Maxie. Finally, her voice answered quietly and it struck me that for the first time ever, Maxie sounded old.

"I understand," she almost whispered. "I just hate it."

"Me, too. Get some rest. I will call you tomorrow."

"Okay, I will try. I love you."

"Me, too."

I checked my phone messages. Matt, Marlo, Ava, and Mutt had called. Only Matt's call was returned.

"Maxie will be fine," I lied.

Maxie would never be fine with Matt's choice, but for now Matt needed to hear these words. With certainty and good reason, he and I knew that she'd repeatedly make her anger known. To reassure her with words we barely believed would be hard.

The day had been full of contrasts. An afternoon filled with the harmless banter and gentle flirtation between two old friends had mutated into an emotional breakdown when Matt told me of his choice to serve in the Armed Forces.

My pride in his commitment had nothing to do with my fear for his safety. I was furious that the world had deteriorated to the point where we needed to be on the alert and have our children protect us.

I was a mess, tense, sore, and stiff. My body felt as if it'd been pounded with a heavy mallet. With the hope that a bath would help me relax, I turned on the hot water, pulled off my clothes, and sunk into the bathwater before it'd reached the rim of the tub.

Helpless to protect my child, I was sadder and more afraid than ever. To the four walls of my bathroom, I screamed, "You will not take my child. You will not hurt him." Then I pulled my knees up close to my chest, put my head down between them, and began to weep.

My medications demanded that I do my best to rest and relax, but yesterday's turmoil had left me little time to do so. Without having slept the night before, the next day at work stretched long and thin.

Oblivious to my limited concentration, my young students continued to engage each other with their natural inquisitiveness. At the end of the school day, I went home, turned off my phone and crashed into bed. It was three thirty. Four hours later I came to and walked into the kitchen, hungry for nothing important.

My attraction to food preparation was minimal. No longer responsible to demonstrate healthy food choices to Matthew, I cobbled together nourishment without guilt, spicy chips, lemons, hot sauce and sharp-tasting salsa. A cold glass of leftover sake washed it all down.

A check of my phone indicated that messages waited. Without surprise, Maxie accounted for three of the calls. Mutt was logged in at two, and Matthew one.

In reverse order, Matthew's call was answered first. With no one at home, my message, "I'll speak to you tomorrow. Kiss Jodi. I love you," would do.

Maxie was next.

Unusually subdued, she said quietly, "You needed time to think. Are you better?"

My answer was a truthful, "No."

She replied, "Me, too."

To encourage myself more than she, I replied weakly, "Maxie, Matthew will be okay."

"Okay. I'm beat and did nothing all day but worry." The sound of her fiddling with her ever-present charm bracelets was a distant reminder of my once normal life.

"Please try to get some rest, or you'll get sick."

"Okay," she said. "You're a great mother."

"So are you, Maxie."

The certainty of our shared history dictated that we would continue to tumble over each other's fears, and then lift each other up until we collided against each other again.

It was time to call Mutt, but the phone rang and interrupted my dialing. It was he. Ripping mad, he shouted, "Are you alright? Did we have too nice a time together on Sunday? You disappeared and I was worried. Tell me what's going on."

Mutt's well-meant words kicked hard against me. With great speed the world and my life had changed, but where to start? Was it cancer, was it September 11, or was it Matthew? Was it just the confluence of life's capriciousness?

Pressured, I raised my voice and roared back at him, "Matthew may be going to the Persian Gulf."

"What the hell are you talking about?" Mutt shouted back.

"Mutt, I'm both proud and scared for him. If something happens to him..."

Mutt interrupted me mid-sentence and repeated, "What are you talking about?"

"Matthew's enlisted in the Coast Guard. He may be going to the Persian Gulf."

Mutt hesitated for a moment, then said, "Oh my. Do you want me to come over and keep you company?"

It was a kind, generous offer, but he would have distracted me as I re-evaluated my feelings.

"No, thank you. I'm not ready for company, even you."

There was a long silence. Waiting for him to start shouting again, I looked out the bedroom window at trees in the garden next door. Their leaves had already begun to dry and fade.

"All right, Baby Girl," Mutt answered with forced calmness. "I understand. I'm here if you need me."

"I know, Mutt, I know."

Relieved to be off the phone, I fixed myself a drink. Adding some tonic and lemon made it all the more perfect, but I'd forgotten to buy cranberry juice to make it spectacularly complete.

Tomorrow I would buy some cranberry juice and damn it, by tomorrow, I'd best be in control of my feelings, or be at risk to become worthless to myself and anyone else.

Holding my drink, I walked into the den and put my glass on a table. With both hands, I pulled albums filled with pictures of Matthew from a closet, laid them next to my drink, and sat down on the couch.

Matthew had been a sunny, outgoing, personable child who'd always relished singular adventures. Summer camp rapidly converted into more dramatic escapades. Mountaineering, expeditions, sky diving, and solo trekking in Africa for eight months had been just a few of his adventures. At the start of each journey, Matthew bubbled with excitement as I tried to control my maternal fears and remember these were his choices to make and his challenges to master.

Skimming through these pictures was an emotional feast to be savored. I prayed that Matthew would make a lifetime of his own memories, each to be safeguarded and revisited as he chose.

With my drink refilled, I returned to my bedroom, looked at the clock, and realized it was well past ten o'clock.

After a quick shower, I dried off, got back into bed, and reached for my pills. With a deep sip of my cocktail, I swallowed one pill, then two, and rested my back against the firm pillows. Feeling calmer at last, I was ready to do as Mutt had often suggested: reflect, regroup and restart my emotional engine.

With eyes closed, I admitted that although I'd never believed that my cancer either protected me from the selfishness of others or entitled me to anything at all, on some level I'd hoped that it would act as an offering, something I'd given up to the universe that would shield those I loved from harm.

The carnage of September 11 made me realize that the life one lived counted for little when disaster struck. However, one's life counted as it was lived.

Matthew deserved my support. No matter what my reservations were, my focus needed to be on him. My decision made, I finished my drink, turned off the light, and slept until the next morning.

Having reached an emotional truce within myself, I would do my best to stay positive, although I understood that my susceptibility to life's uncontrollable permutations would make this difficult to sustain.

My need to be close to my family and friends propelled me into their circle of comfort during the months following Matthew's enlistment. However, this respite was transient and could not erase my concern for Matthew's conceivable deployment to the Persian Gulf.

Within weeks, Matthew had breezed through basic training and was now a Petty Officer, First Class, Public Affairs Specialist assigned to the U.S. Coast Guard, Public Affairs Detachment, New York.

Shortly after, he volunteered to serve in the Persian Gulf for at least half a year, and in December 2003, it was time for him to leave.

CHAPTER THIRTY-ONE

Not Summer Camp

Matthew and I alone drove to the airport so he could board his overseas flight. Jodi and he had said their goodbyes the night before. I wished hard for the traffic to slow us down, or for any relatively safe delay that would cause Matt to miss his plane. Better still, perhaps I could stay on the highway and make a run to Canada and hide him there.

But the roads were clear. We didn't get a flat tire, run out of gas, or suffer any calamity that I'd wished for. Instead, there was Matt with his unshakeable resolve and no way that he would agree to do anything but make his connections to get to the Middle East.

Our goodbye was long and painful, without any small talk.

When the time came for us to part, tears rushed from my eyes and poured down my checks as I clung to him. I double-kissed each of his checks and whispered, "Be safe my son. I love you. Come home."

"Mom, I'll be all right. Just take care of Jodi."

"I will. I love you."

"I love you, too."

He stepped back and lifted one of his two large duffel bags onto one shoulder and leaned down and picked up the other bag with his free hand, then walked into the terminal. As I watched him all but disappear into the crowd, he stopped, put down one of his bags and turned back to face me.

For an instant I thought he'd changed his mind and was going to come back home with me, but instead he smiled and waved, then picked up his bag and walked away.

I started to walk back to my parked car but took only a few steps before I stopped. For support, I leaned against a nearby pillar, doubled over, and cried.

Within minutes, I felt a strong arm move around my waist as a deep voice said close to my ear, "Mother, your son will be all right."

Confused and frightened, my body pulled up and away from the stranger. I lifted my head and saw a short, broad-shouldered man with an angular face and brown skin. He wore the uniform of an airport policeman.

"I'm sorry to have frightened you," he said, "but I watched you say goodbye to your son. I saw how upset you were and thought you might collapse."

"Thank you," I answered. "I don't know if I'm strong enough to deal with his choice to go."

He replied softly, "One day at a time, just one day at a time. That's what I try to do. My son's been overseas for almost a year."

My return trip from the airport was awful. It was hard to believe that I'd just left Matthew there and he would begin his travel to Bahrain. Mentally, I would suspend my breath until he returned home safe.

Without question, I would pray endlessly to not outlive my child as so many mothers and fathers were forced to do as the result of the horrors of September 11.

On that dreadful day, Matthew had climbed the steps up from the subway beneath lower Manhattan only to find that he'd ridden into hell.

He watched the flames, smelled the smoke, and witnessed those who, in their futile attempts to escape the mortally wounded Twin Towers, tragically leaped to their deaths.

Covered in ash, he and thousands of others had slowly made their way home across the Brooklyn Bridge. Forever changed by the day's insanity, he was compelled to respond to this despicable act of hate and enlisted in the United States Coast Guard Reserve.

Crushed together, my feelings twisted and turned inward. Tears blurred my vision and forced me to pull to the side of the highway and stop my car. Within seconds I collapsed over the steering wheel and began to weep.

Tearful, I called Jodi. On the first ring she answered my call. "Did he really leave? Is he gone?"

I hated to say "yes," but it was true. Matthew had gone. I heard her catch her breath and then sadly exhale it in defeat.

I asked, "Would you like me to visit with you?"

She sighed, hesitated for a minute, and then said softly, "Thank you, but I need to pull myself together." She paused for a moment, and then asked gently, "I know this is going to be hard for you, too. Let's have dinner tomorrow. I'm not working."

"Agreed. If you need me, call me at any time," I replied.

"Okay," she whispered.

As I replayed my goodbye to Matthew and wondered if we would ever see him again, the sadness I felt was unlike anything I'd experienced.

To call Maxie would be pointless. With almost reassuring comfort, she'd played diva and had taken refuge in her bed before Matthew's departure. Unable to face him, she'd said her goodbyes on the telephone.

Inherently resilient, Maxie would rebound, but as she missed Matthew more and more each day, for her not to lash out in frustration at anyone near would be her test.

The blast of an eighteen-wheeler's horn snapped me to attention. The clock on my car's dashboard showed me I'd been sitting in my car for almost an hour and a half. It also told me that Matthew's plane had already left and that as each minute passed, he moved still farther away.

Tomorrow would not be a better day, but it would be one day closer to Matthew's homecoming.

Wiped out and feeling utterly useless, I wanted to mimic Maxie and disappear under my bed covers to dull my feelings. Restarting my car, I pulled onto the highway and drove home. In less time than expected I reached my street, where I saw a familiar, well-traveled, white BMW convertible parked across from the entrance to my garage. It belonged to Mutt.

Damn, I thought, why was he here now?

He knew I'd taken Matthew to the airport that morning. While parked at the roadside, I'd listened to his messages. With each call he'd become more anxious, more agitated. The urgency in his voice had stopped me cold, but too upset by Matthew's leaving, I'd let his calls go unanswered.

Obviously he needed to be here and reach out to me, but rather than feel relieved I felt pressured, as if he'd invaded my private space and wanted me to navigate his feelings at a time when I could barely steady mine.

I reversed my car to the left and backed out of the street. I turned right at the next corner and parked my car so that I could calm down and think.

Mutt had always been my champion, and I was content to be his beloved friend. As a witness to my many falls from grace, Mutt knew my secrets. Throughout it all, he remained nonjudgmental and propelled me forward with confidence. Since my mastectomies, my life had taken many turns, but it was clear that he and I had grown closer. More than once we'd mimed the dance of lovers, but not wanting to risk the loss of our friendship, we'd resisted the play.

Consumed by the ongoing drama of my life, I'd successfully avoided sorting out my feelings for him, but somehow I believed that a resolution was near. Perhaps hidden somewhere deep was my fear that it might signal the end to our friendship.

I shook my head, cleaned my face with a small generic wipe, then switched on my car's engine, put my foot down lightly on the gas pedal, and moved ahead so that by the time my cell phone rang again, my car was stopped alongside Mutt's. Sensing my presence, he looked up, put his cell phone down, and smiled.

My answer was a tentative nod of my head.

After I'd parked my car, we met in my lobby. Smartly dressed in all black, he leaned against the side of the elevator door and looked directly at me. Without a word I walked past him into the waiting elevator. He followed close behind me, and within minutes after we'd closed my front door behind us, Mutt pulled me into his arms.

I responded to his warmth and began to cry.

For me, it had been an awful day, one almost beyond repair. Unbidden, Mutt's presence had initially been an unwanted intrusion, but at least with Mutt here I felt less alone. How could I have not wanted him with me?

Within seconds, my tears turned into sobs. Wordlessly, he pressed me even closer to his chest and stroked my head. The warmth of his hands suspended my thoughts as he caressed me, no longer as a friend but as a lover. Lifting my eyes to meet his, I saw only love and compassion.

We found our way into my bedroom and lay down together on the bed. As we slowly turned to each other, I mutely ruminated over my scared body and wondered how I would respond to him.

Shyness overcame me. Would my scars matter? Would he compare me to other women who hadn't been carved up and stitched back together? Would it all be so strangely different that I wouldn't relax and enjoy the intimacy?

Mutt pulled me close and the uncertainty fell away. As we crossed the boundary of friends to lovers, he kissed my scars with tenderness. It was almost as if this intimate moment had been earned; the sorrow, trauma, loss, soul searching, rebuilding, and healing gave a reason to seek sanctuary. For the first time in ages, I felt safe.

Later, as he slept, I traced my finger along the scar stretching the length of his beautiful body. Created from 150 stitches, it was the sacred marker of his bypass surgery.

Beginning at his collarbone, I glided slowly down along the middle of his chest. Resting for a moment, I placed my head upon his thigh, and continued along his leg, stopping at his ankle. I gave thanks that he was alive. Soon after, I fell asleep close by his side, fulfilled.

Much later in the day, the ring of my telephone woke us. My first thought was that something had happened to Matthew, and I rushed to lift the receiver. I heard Jodi's soft voice at the other end.

She asked, "Could you please come and stay with me for a little while? I don't want to be alone."

"I'll be there within the hour," was my answer.

Wide awake, Mutt sat up in bed. We looked at each other and smiled as I kissed him on his check.

He stroked my face and whispered, "I love you more than you will ever know."

I hugged him and then rushed into the bathroom to shower. When I re-entered my bedroom, Mutt had already dressed and was ready to leave.

As he watched me, I stopped dressing and walked to him. With his face now held between my hands, I kissed him lightly on his lips and whispered, "Thank you for being my friend."

He reached his arms around my back and pulled me close against his chest. He sighed, and I sensed it was from resignation that I still thought of him as "friend."

As I retreated from his embrace, he stood up and rested his arm around my shoulder. After we'd walked to the front door, he turned me to face him. "All I want is to be close to you. I hate leaving you alone and being without you."

Why now, I thought. Why now when my life was such a mess did Mutt want more from me than I felt I could give?

Intuitively he voiced my reservation. "Let's make no promises and just see what happens. I'll try to make no demands. Just try."

Without giving him the answer he wanted, I kissed him goodbye and closed the door. For a few minutes thereafter, I remained still and tried to digest what had just materialized between Mutt and me.

For so long, he and I had been so good at being each other's dear, dear friends; to change that would be difficult, as I was now consumed with both my son's well-being and trying to inch my way back to better health.

A deeper relationship with Mutt, or anyone else, was not something I could imagine at this point, because it would require both time and energy; neither of which I had.

My wish was that our friendship would survive, but my immediate concern was to dress quickly and meet Jodi.

Jodi looked terrible. Her misery was painfully apparent as tears still covered her face. I reached my arms up and hugged her tight. Then I broke down and began to weep. We held each other for longer than I can remember, long enough to combine in our love and prayers for Matthew.

Breaking free from each other, Jodi looked down at me and said, "Thank you for coming."

I replied, "Thank you for asking me to be with you. You're my link to Matthew. You're not alone."

After another warm hug, we separated to wash our faces. Although we remained anxious and drained, afterward we decided to go out to eat and drink to Matthew's safe and speedy return.

From that evening forward, Jodi and I spoke regularly and often met for dinner, drinks, or a movie. Each of us tried to be strong for the other, although we knew that neither of us felt that way. Nonetheless, we struggled together to make the best of a difficult situation.

Maxie had gotten out of bed the day after Matthew left and called me to see if his departure went smoothly. In reality, what she needed was my confirmation that Matthew had indeed defied her wishes and left the country.

"Well," she said with obvious sarcasm, "you raised an independent child. It's not enough that Matthew had to go climb mountains and almost scare me to death, but now that he has gone off to the Middle East, he will surely kill me."

How could I disagree with her when I felt the same way? Rather than defend Matthew's right to do as he wished, I surprised her with my answer. "Maxie, you are absolutely right."

Stunned by my response, she asked, "You agree with me?"

"Yes, Maxie, I do."

"Marjorie, I miss him."

"Me, too, Maxie, me, too."

In the months that followed, Maxie did try her best to be patient and kind to Jodi and me, but Maxie would not have been Maxie if she'd failed to more often than not go on a rip, angry that she'd not stopped Matthew from going away.

CHAPTER THIRTY-TWO

Return 2

When Jodi, Maxie, or I received a call from Matthew, we'd share what little news we had and answer the other's anxious questions. "How did he sound? Is he all right? What can we send to him? Where is he now?"

We knew that he was exhausted and seemed to work 24/7. Only after the fact did we learn that Matthew had served in Basra, Iraq, Yemen, and Kuwait, all of which caused us to breathe deeper and pray even harder.

Jodi seemed to lose herself in her work and labored many hours a week. I worried about her but held my advice; she needed to manage her life as she saw fit.

Mutt and I continued to communicate, but saw each other less frequently as it became obvious that I could not shift closer to him. At times I wondered what would have been if, years earlier, we would have gambled on our feelings and made those promises one can only make when young. Without a doubt, some of them would have been kept, but more would have been broken, which would have tested our bonds or done irreparable harm.

As friends, we'd remained close but not responsible for the other's happiness. Perhaps we'd loved each other too much to become less to each other than we imagined. Or perhaps we'd simply been cowards, each too needy to set the other free.

Mutt's feelings mattered to me, and I took no pleasure in not responding to him as he wished. It was no less painful to our relationship for Mutt and me to gradually retreat from each other, but far more respectful of it than to subject it to continuous disappointment.

Maxie did her best to keep busy. Her support of people with disabilities was tireless. She was a vocal advocate for them all her life, and she tirelessly fought for their dignity and their right to be given the opportunities to thrive and develop.

In the past, she and I had joined together to plan fundraisers. Many of our trips to Atlantic City were opportunities for us to conference and orchestrate our next project. She waited for me to get stronger so we could undertake another event, but still insisted that I go with her to Atlantic City.

"Marjorie, let's go this Saturday morning. I have the driver, and we can just relax all the way. I have some ideas for a new project. I need your input. You need the sea air."

"Maxie, I love your rationalization. We are in the casino all day, and the only time we breathe sea air is walking to and from the car."

She laughed and said, "True, but it's better than nothing. Let's go have some fun. I can't stand being home. I think too much about your crazy son who'll surely kill me with worry."

"Okay, Maxie, let's go."

Sometimes she would add, "Would Jodi like to come?"

Without the heart to tell her that Jodi didn't gamble and that her occasional trip with Matthew to a racetrack was more a reason for her to dress up than bet, I fudged, "That's sweet, but Jodi is working. Let's take her to dinner this week instead."

Often Maxie would be beside herself with worry and twisted into such a knot that she would be all but inconsolable. Unable to hold her feelings in check, she spat out words I dared not speak.

"Marjorie, I am done with all this waiting to hear from your son. No one has heard from him in weeks. Is he still alive?"

It was painful for me to hear her verbalize my concerns, and I wished at times that she would keep these feelings locked inside her, as if speaking them might render them true. But, sympathetic to her need to express her fears, and to avoid confrontation, I would hold my tongue and answer simply, "Maxie, I'm worried, too. I have no answer. Let's just hope for the best."

Those conversations left me anxious and frightened. Short and to the point, they managed to cut through to my heart. Until Matthew's next call I worried nonstop. Time did nothing but make the present more tenuous. With every death of one of our troops I realized how quickly we were losing our children over there, and felt all the more discouraged at not being able to intervene and end the bloodshed.

For me, each day had its own pulse anchored by work and medicine, and for the most part I continued to get stronger emotionally and physically. Cancer remained a concern, but at this point it had become the acknowledged but unwanted guest who sat in the corner of the room waiting for the worst to happen.

Less tired, and now seeing the oncologist at six-month intervals, I began to exercise with more regularity and less fatigue. My chest muscles had healed and with effort I resumed playing tennis, but understandably, my first attempt was limited to a strained half hour. After weeks of hard work, I succeeded in playing a full hour with a smile on my face.

As winter moved into a welcomed spring, I started to ride my bicycle again. A few labored blocks over time became ten easy miles. It felt great to be outside and moving along at a modest but steady pace.

Although it took me days to recover from each of my physical activities, I was empowered.

Ava and I played with her son and often walked with him to a local park. For me to be able to hold him was a joy, something I had waited to do since my surgery. Marlo and I were back on track, sharing time doing small things and laughing about nothing in particular. Once again we began to make plans for a weekend away, predicated on Matthew's return in June.

Throughout New York City one could still see some of the now torn and faded pictures of loved ones lost in the attacks. They never failed to remind me of the bereaved mother who had collapsed in my arms, exhausted from her futile search for her son. Without her child, I could only imagine her intolerable grief. Ground Zero remained an ugly reminder of our vulnerability. Mired in bureaucratic red tape, it would take years before insurance claims were settled and a plan to rebuild the area was agreed upon that would reflect our city's resilience and provide a respectful memorial to the lives lost on September 11, 2001. Nonetheless, people continued to be drawn to the site, all of them eager to personally reflect and mourn this tragedy.

During this time, for me to say that I missed the companionship of a man would not be accurate. I was still recovering from my beat down from breast cancer and preoccupied with Matthew's trials. But having enjoyed the loving, wonderful experience of making love with Mutt, I felt confident that with luck, there would an opportunity for me to connect with someone and build a sound relationship.

Cancer, 9/11 and Matthew's deployment had combined to act as a mandate to live as I saw fit and not settle for anything less than wonderful.

In time, Matthew's expected arrival dwindled down from six months to three months, then two and one, but my excitement to see him was tempered by the knowledge that he was still in harm's way.

Finally with no more days, weeks, or months to count, I received the call from Jodi that Matt was on his way home.

"Marjorie," Jodi said excitedly, "Matthew's on his way back to the United States."

Before she finished, I screamed, "Thank God! I can't believe it! Are you sure? Is he all right? How do you know?"

Jodi laughed and said, "Wait, wait. Take a breath and let me answer you."

Silenced, I held my tongue and listened to her speak as my eyes filled with long-held tears of relief. "Matthew's just called me. He's at the airport in Bahrain and due to leave within the hour. First he will land in Virginia to be debriefed, and soon after he is on a plane home. I can't wait to see him."

"Me, too. I'll call Maxie. I will tell you what she says. It's going to be classic for sure."

I could hear her giggle as she added, "Okay, there is so much for me to do to get the house ready for Matthew's return. I haven't really attended to it for ages."

"Not to worry. I'll be over soon and will help you clean up. I think a good bottle of wine shared between us will help."

"Me, too," she laughed.

Overcome with relief that Matthew was indeed safe and on his way home, after I'd said, "I love you, Jodi," I danced though my home to an imagined tune. Mid-twirl, the thought of Maxie stopped me in place.

I composed myself, dialed her phone number, and said "Hi Maxie, what are you doing?"

Obviously annoyed about something, she muttered, "Not much. I'm bored. Make it quick. I need to shower and get out of the house. I have an appointment in Manhattan and..." She stopped for a moment, and then asked, "Why do you sound so happy?"

I answered slowly so that she would listen to my words. "Well, Maxie, Jodi just called to tell me that Matthew is coming home today."

Shocked, she asked in disbelief, "What did you say? Are you sure? Where is he now? Can I call him? I don't believe you."

With a smile, I said firmly, "Maxie, be quiet. Believe me. Matthew is on his way home."

She caught her breath and murmured, "Thank God," then she added as only Maxie could, "it's about time. What can I do?"

I answered, "Nothing now, but soon enough we'll have a party to plan."

Later that day, I drove to Jodi and Matthew's home. It would be wonderful to see him there again, comfortable, settled, and safe.

Though Jodi and I were nervous wrecks, we opened a fine bottle of wine, turned on some music and cleaned the house alongside Jodi's parents, who'd driven in from Westchester to celebrate Matthew's imminent arrival.

Within hours, Jodi was off to pick up Matthew at the same airport where, six months earlier, I had left him. When she called to say, "I can't believe it. His plane landed, and I see him walking to me. He looks wonderful," I answered, "Thank you. Go to him. Call me later."

My son was alive and home. At that moment I was the luckiest mother in the world, no longer wrapped in a heavy blanket of unhappiness. With bowed head, I prayed first that Matthew and Jodi would never again be faced with such a heart-wrenching separation, and then for the safety and quick return of those children who remained overseas.

My reunion with Matthew was beyond wonderful. He, Jodi, and I met at one of his favorite places for brunch. He saw me first and somehow managed to come up behind me and tap me on my shoulder.

"Excuse me, do you know Matthew Belson?"

"What?" I answered and turned around.

There stood my son. With a wide grin on his face and tears in his eyes he held his arms open to receive my embrace. It was a very good day indeed.

More quiet than usual, I sat through the meal simply content to just watch and listen to the exchanges between Matthew and Jodi again. Seeing them together filled me with hope for their future. Warm and loving, they reminded me of the young lovers they'd been before September 11 had crashed into their world.

Undoubtedly, it would take time for them to reacquaint and restart their marriage, but they'd survived the worst and would move ahead together.

Matthew said, "I'm glad to have served my country. I'm glad to be home. I missed you all very much."

In time, Matthew would share experiences with me as he wished. My sense was that some things were best left unsaid, and with that I was more than satisfied.

Later, I called Mutt to tell him of Matthew's return. "How are you, Baby Girl? I've missed you," drenched me with warmth. I felt myself answering him naturally. "Mutt, I've missed you, too. Matthew's come safely home."

He answered, "Thank God. I haven't stopped praying for him, you know."

I nodded to myself and said, "I knew that you would."

Then he asked, "How about you and me celebrating his return? Let's go to Azul."

I thought for a moment before answering, "I will let you know when."

As expected, with patience he replied, "All in good time, Baby Girl, all in good time."

Matthew's welcome home party was held later in the month. It was close to his birthday, so friends and family joined in a dual celebration. As drinks were downed and toasts made, all of us gave thanks for the miracle of a life spared.

Maxie and Matthew had their private reunion days before. She'd cried and railed at him, "Matthew, if you ever go off like that again, I'm absolutely finished with you."

We laughed and noted that while the English said, "God save the queen," we'd instead learned to say, "God save Maxie."

For Matthew's party, Maxie spared nothing. Dressed in Louis Feraud splendor as if she were going to a fine cocktail party; her evening suit was smart and deep blue. With matching shoes and evening bag, she looked happy and vibrant. She paid no mind that the event was held in a favored local bar. It was a party, and a party she would have.

It was fun to watch her mingle with the guests. To all who would listen, she complained at high speed about her first-born grandson's adventures.

"What the hell was he thinking? He has to be crazy. I hate him and his mother. She was crazy to let him go off all these years. If I didn't love them both so much, I would disown them. Poor Jodi. She married into this crazy family."

When she was finished spewing forth, she would invariably wink at either me or Matthew and smile.

At one point late into the evening Maxie turned to me and said in a low, conspiratorial voice, "Okay, enough. The food is terrible, my feet hurt, and I need to go home and eat something decent. Do you want to go to Atlantic City with me tomorrow?"

I felt a wide smile coming on and couldn't quit grinning as I scanned the room. It was almost a cliché, but the most beloved people in my world all stood within a few feet of one another. We were safe.

"Atlantic City tomorrow or not?" Maxie put a hand on her hip.

As I burst out in laughter, life never felt so good. Maxie stood her ground with a frown. I smiled and finally asked, "What time do we leave?"

CPSIA information can be obtained at www.ICGtesting.com
Printed in the USA
BVOW03s1609150914

366817BV00001B/2/P